THE SHAPE WE ...

SARAH BOSELEY is the health editor of the *Guardian* newspaper, writing about health and medical issues with both a UK and a global perspective for the last 15 years. She has won ten awards for her work, including the One World Media award (twice), the BMJ Group journalism award and the Lorenzo Natali prize from the European Commission. She has two daughters and lives in London. @sarahboseley

THE SHAPE WE'RE IN

How Junk Food and Diets
Are Shortening Our Lives

SARAH BOSELEY

First published in 2014
by Guardian Books,
Kings Place, 90 York Way, London N1 9GU
and Faber & Faber Ltd,
Bloomsbury House, 74–77 Great Russell Street, London WC1B 3DA

Printed and bound in Great Britain by CPI Group (UK) Ltd, Croydon, CR0 4YY

A CIP record for this book is available from the British Library

ISBN 978–1783–3503–84

Designed and set by seagulls.net

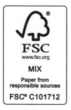

FSC
www.fsc.org
MIX
Paper from
responsible sources
FSC® C101712

2 4 6 8 10 9 7 5 3 1

*To my mum and dad, who grew up
in a very different world from this one.*

CONTENTS

I went into a McDonald's yesterday and said, 'I'd like some fries.' The girl at the counter said, 'Would you like some fries with that?'

Jay Leno

PROLOGUE

I did not really understand why obesity was such a problem until a doctor on the front line, working in Mississippi in the epicentre of the United States' epidemic, showed me some MRI scans of the insides of seriously overweight people's bodies. It was as if fat had been poured into all the gaps and cracks between the organs, a great bulging mass of white on the image. The liver was swollen to a huge size, but the kidneys had been squashed small by the strangulating mass of fat. The diaphragm and lungs had been pushed up into the top of the body and the heart was under pressure. Small surprise, he remarked, if people are breathless.

It was like something from a sci-fi film.

If people knew what this fat was doing to the inside of their bodies, they would surely feel differently about their weight and see it as a more urgent problem than they mostly do. It's not about how you look. It's about what is happening to your insides. We need to think of it like cancer: you can't see what it's doing, but it's doing you real harm.

1

WE ARE ALL IN DENIAL

In May 2012, fire engines, police and an ambulance were called to the family home of a teenager called Georgia Davis in Aberdare, south Wales, in order to get her out of it. Nobody could dream up a more horrifying and humiliating nightmare for a girl of her age. A team of over 40 people was involved in demolishing an upstairs wall of the semi-detached house and constructing a wooden bridge to get a specially reinforced stretcher into her bedroom. Georgia weighed 400kg (63 stone), said some tabloid newspaper reports, while others said 350kg (56 stone). Nobody really knew – she was too heavy at that point to get on the scales. Her rescuers had the delicacy to put up tarpaulins to shield her from the camera lenses as they extracted her through a 10-foot square hole in the brickwork and took her to hospital. She was covered by a sheet, because she could no longer get into any of her clothes.

The 19-year-old was morbidly obese and her organs were failing. Her mother, Lesley, had called the ambulance because she could no longer stand up. For some months she had not moved from her bedroom, where she spent her days on her laptop and watching TV. Eventually, like Alice in Wonderland inside the little house after drinking something she shouldn't, she grew too big to get out of the door.

Unfortunately this was not one of Lewis Carroll's charming Victorian fantasies. It is a true and desperate story of our modern age. Georgia is the extreme marker of a massive problem that has its roots in the way we live today and that affects all of us. Two-thirds of us are overweight. A quarter of us are obese and in real danger of damaging our health and dying prematurely. But we are in denial. Obesity looks like Georgia, we think. It doesn't look like us.

Obesity is a life-shortening condition. Life expectancy, which has risen steadily since records began, may for the first time be about to fall. Moderate obesity cuts life expectancy by two to four years and severe obesity could wipe an entire decade off your life, said the *Lancet* in 2009. The costs to health services and to the world's economies of vast numbers of people becoming sick and unable to work are already huge and increasing. The National Heath Service is spending £5 billion a year treating heart attacks, strokes, diabetes, cancers, liver failure, hip and knee joint problems and other consequences of obesity, and the bill is expected to reach £15 billion within a few decades. Every country has the same soaring costs.[1]

But like an iceberg, only the tip of the problem is yet showing. Obesity began to take off in the 1980s. The full health impact is not yet apparent. The National Audit Office estimated that there were over 30,000 premature deaths and

18 million days of sickness absence caused by obesity in England per year back in 1998. Those numbers must have soared, but no further official count has been done.

With such costs and casualties, you might think we would be on a war-footing with the issue by now. But the reluctance of politicians, the affluent and those who have never had a weight issue to believe that it is about anything other than individual greed, sloth and personal responsibility means that obesity and its health and financial consequences continue to inflict more and more damage. There are a few sporadic initiatives, but no military-scale strategy to reverse it and no general in charge of the campaign.

Indeed, nobody wants ownership of the problem. The humiliation of Georgia tells us much about the reasons why. Most people today are overweight but, they say to themselves, they have nothing whatsoever in common with her. They believe a spell on a diet or a few months of hard work at the gym will sort out the surplus pounds – and yet, somehow, it doesn't. Magazines and newspapers still feature thin women and muscled men as the norm, even though people who look like that are very much a minority. Fatness has become so ordinary that we cease to notice it in the people we meet and don't think of it as an issue for ourselves. When we do, we are divided about the causes and the solutions and those divisions are exploited by those who can make money out of our appetite, inactivity and eventual panicked attempts to lose weight. Meanwhile we turn our face away from extreme cases like Georgia's. If she is what obesity looks like, then the rest of us don't have a problem.

Georgia's troubles were served up as entertainment in the tabloids, which paid her for the story, as if she were part of a freak show. In photographs (and there are many), her face, above the mountain of flesh, is curiously passive. The expressionless look reminds me of a painting in the Wellcome Collection of a 36-year-old man called Daniel Lambert, painted in the early 1800s. He weighed 320kg (50 stone) and exhibited himself to the curious in an apartment in Piccadilly, London, for a shilling a time. Poor Georgia is not Alice, in a bit of a fix and unable to straighten her arm without putting it out of the window. She is the Elephant Man, whose appearance evokes pity and horror – in this case, mixed with condemnation. The newspapers offer Georgia's story as a sort of modern morality tale and the unspoken but implicit judgment on her is that she is the epitome of greed.

There is little sympathy either for Paul Mason from Ipswich, who is said to have once been the world's fattest man. Mason lost 292kg (46 stone) of his 444kg (70 stone) after gastric-band surgery and posed for photographs with his skin hanging loose like so much empty sacking – another exhibition piece from the fat freak show.

Neither young women like Georgia nor men like Mason are to be found at middle-class dinner parties where the influential gather – the opinion-formers, be they lawyers, bankers, journalists or businesspeople, who set agendas with and for the politicians. They will be disgusted but unmoved by the naked photos that Mason posed for in the desperate hope of advancing his case for plastic surgery. The reaction to the pictures is most commonly not one of sympathy or understanding but revulsion, coupled with anger that he should propose to burden the NHS still further.

It is the same in the United States, where obesity itself is so prevalent and yet the word is applied only to the very extreme cases. These are people to gawp at. Take Michael Hebranko, dubbed the world's biggest yo-yo dieter as if this was only about slimming. Hebranko, from Staten Island, New York, says he once had a good career in a pharmaceutical company as well as a happy marriage and a son – so not such a loser. Yet he has twice weighed 500kg (80 stone). In 1990, he made the *Guinness Book of Records* for the greatest ever weight loss – 420kg (66 stone). But it all went back on.

'I know eating is killing me,' said Hebranko to the Huffington Post in March 2012. 'I am a food addict, just like an alcoholic or a heroin addict. I've been told all my life if I kept eating I wouldn't make it to the age of 60. Now that birthday is just two years away and doctors don't think I'll make it. They told me in September I had congestive heart failure, liver failure and kidney failure. My wife, Madelaine, and I have been told to put our affairs in order.'

It is easy for most people, even if obese themselves, to dismiss Georgia's and Hebranko's sufferings as nothing to do with them. These are just grotesque individuals with no self-control. They are lazy, feckless, hopeless people – and not like us. Never mind that Hebranko was once a success story and Georgia is very young. Obesity, we think, means somebody huge who can hardly walk, incapable of living a normal life.

7

Except it doesn't. The more the problem has spread, the more it has disappeared from view. There are many obese people around us whom we don't even notice. We may look like them ourselves. Overweight and obese bodies have become normalised. Our minds have become attuned to fleshy people. Look at photographs from the 1950s and 60s. They resemble collections of stick people from a Lowry painting. The children in their baggy shorts seem malnourished. You can even see ribs in those who play on the beach. But in fact, most of these are people of a healthy weight.

Experiments have shown that what we now think is normal is actually overweight and even obese. Researchers asked nearly 1000 men and 1000 women their weight, height and how they would describe themselves on a scale from 'very underweight' to 'obese' in 1999. They then repeated the exercise eight years later. In 2007, the people weighed dramatically more but fewer realised it. Only 75 per cent correctly considered themselves overweight, compared to 81 per cent eight years earlier.[2] We just don't see it. We don't want to see it. So we reject Georgia as if her experiences have nothing to tell us about ourselves.

Yet Georgia was just a child when it all got out of hand and could hardly be held to blame for her weight at that time. She was 15 when she first hit the front page of the *Sun*, weighing over 200kg (33 stone) and branded Britain's fattest teen. The question everybody eagerly asked was what had she been eating – how big a mountain of food, how many cakes at one sitting, how many kebabs and burgers? Why she should want to was very much of subsidiary interest. Georgia and her mother Lesley, who is also obese, spoke of comfort eating after Georgia's dad died when she was five. In later stories it emerged that before she was 10, she had become the carer of both Lesley, who had heart disease, and her stepfather Arthur Treloar. Social services discussed removing her from the family, but she resisted. By any stretch of the imagination, Georgia had a tough childhood.

We can avoid overweight by exercising personal responsibility, say politicians, voicing the script written by the food industry. We choose what we put into our mouths. We ought to know what will make us fat and have the self-restraint to stop eating. But can you really make that judgment of Georgia at the age of seven, who even then weighed 70kg (11 stone) and whom Lesley admits she fed with condensed milk as a baby, weaning her onto tinned potatoes and later filling her up with fried eggs and chips? If not, because most people would surely blame the parents rather than the child, then when does it become Georgia's fault that she is fat – at 19, still a teenager, when heavy lifting gear was required to remove her from her house, or at 20, or 30?

Tabloid journalist Susie Boniface, then writing anonymously as *Mirror* online blogger Fleet Street Fox, did attempt to address this very conundrum in May 2012, on the day after Georgia was rescued from her house, but you can see how she labours to keep her readers with her. Don't skip to the next story, she is implicitly saying – I feel as disgusted by obese people as you do, but children are a special case.

'I've no time for fat people,' she writes. She is not referring to those who are carrying a few extra stone, she claims, before continuing:

'I'm talking about the truly, appallingly obese. The ones who eat so much they're going to cause everyone else problems – the ones who scoff their way up the NHS waiting lists, who can't work because of their size, whose very existence takes money and time and effort and sympathy out of society and gives nothing at all back – them I just can't stand.'

They should sort themselves out and not expect the state to help, she writes, making us complicit with her judgment:

'That's how many of us think. We see a fatty and feel scornful, presuming they're just too bone idle and greedy, and we push past their waddling forms on the way to somewhere we won't have to look at them.'

But even if the quarter of adults in the population who are obese deserve this opprobrium, what about the children, she then asks. And she tells how Georgia sold her story to the tabloids and TV to get the money to go to a weight-loss camp in North Carolina where she lost half her bodyweight, then how she came back to find nothing had changed at home – her mother bought fish and chips because there was nothing to eat in the house. She quoted Georgia's own account:

'Around eight weeks after returning from camp I drifted off the plan. I felt really alone. My parents weren't doing it with me at home and my friends weren't doing it at college so there was no motivation to continue.

'I started reverting to my old ways. I wouldn't eat for half a day then start bingeing into the night. I knew things were getting out of control but I didn't want to return to the US because I missed my family too much and I was desperate to go to college and be a normal teenager.'

Georgia, Boniface declaims, has been let down by her parents and by the state – and, she apparently reluctantly concludes, those morbidly obese adults that she finds so disgusting may have once been children like her too:

'Fat adults often have complex eating disorders and need psychiatric treatment before any physical improvement can take place because they're self-abusing – but they don't get any. They should, rather than being shoved past and ignored by people. There's still a bit of me that thinks they could start by just laying off the cake. But fat children on the other hand are the victims of the adults they rely upon to look after them … It's about time we turned that revulsion we feel for the morbidly obese into proper social change, passed laws to make our food healthier and take action when children are being let down.'

This brave reasoning did not persuade another *Mirror* columnist writing about obesity less than a year later. Carole Malone in January 2013 reflected the more popular line, which we are also constantly offered by politicians and the food industry. She said she was fed up with the excuses: 'While I know that in these PC times taking responsibility for my own body is a novel concept, the facts are undeniable. If you exercise more and eat less, you lose weight. Which is why I'm furious at the suggestion that all obese people are hopeless "addicts" who are somehow rendered powerless in the face of a chip butty or a jumbo pizza.'

Malone said she was 82kg (13 stone) and technically obese herself but knew it was her own fault.

She continued: 'The only way people ever get thin – and stay thin – is when they want to and when they're prepared to put in the work to make it happen.'

The first stories about Georgia ran in August 2008, less than a year after the seminal Foresight report into obesity was published, commissioned by the Labour government. This two-year investigation by an independent expert team did not lay blame on individuals like Georgia, and tell them just to stop eating. It said that the causes of obesity were 'embedded in an extremely complex biological system, set within an equally complex societal framework'. It pointed the finger at what it called our 'obesogenic environment'.

What they meant was the wide availability of cheap, filling, very fattening fast food and sweet drinks that are advertised to us on every street and all the commercial TV stations, together with the cakes, pastries, crisps, snacks, fizzy pop and packaged ready meals sold in the supermarkets. We cannot avoid the displays of biscuits and sweets strategically positioned in the aisles at sight-level or in reach of children at the check-out. Vending machines at sports centres sell high-calorie bars of sweets and drinks that threaten to undo the health benefits of swimming or playing volleyball. We drive rather than take the bus, let alone walk. Recreation is the TV and the computer. We no

longer feel our children are safe playing outside in the park
or on the street.

So it is not just the individual's fault if they put on
weight. Sir David King, the government's chief scientific
adviser and head of the government office for science,
wrote in his introduction that Foresight's findings 'challenge the simple portrayal of obesity as an issue of personal
willpower – eating too much and doing too little'.

It was a problem for the whole of society, said the
report: 'People in the UK today don't have less willpower
and are not more gluttonous than previous generations.
Nor is their biology significantly different to that of their
forefathers. Society, however, has radically altered over the
past five decades, with major changes in work patterns,
transport, food production and food sales. These changes
have exposed an underlying biological tendency, possessed
by many people, to both put on weight and retain it.'

It was putting us all at risk of a whole range of chronic
diseases – those long-term conditions that we cannot
easily get over, unlike flu or measles. They include type
2 diabetes, high blood pressure, heart disease, stroke and
cancer. These diseases can also wreck a person's wellbeing
and quality of life, as well as their ability to hold down a
job and earn a living.

'The pace of the technological revolution is outstripping
human evolution and, for an increasing number of people,
weight gain is the inevitable – and largely involuntary –
consequence of exposure to a modern lifestyle,' King wrote.
'This is not to dismiss personal responsibility altogether, but

to highlight a reality: that the forces that drive obesity are, for many people, overwhelming. Although what we identify in this report as "passive obesity" occurs across all population groups, the socially and economically disadvantaged and some ethnic minorities are more vulnerable.'

Georgia is one of the more vulnerable. Aberdare in south Wales where she grew up, 3.5 miles from Merthyr Tydfil, once thrived on iron and then coal mining, which started to decline after the first world war, with the last pits closing in the 1960s. South Wales has known poverty in the past. When the men were down the pit and women took in washing to try to make ends meet, their children ran waif-like in the streets, in threadbare clothes and malnourished.

Poverty today comes with kebabs and chips. It is not about starvation, but cheap junk food. Poor children are still malnourished but they are increasingly overweight. Obesity is allied to a lack of education, low-paid or no paid work and an absence of prospects or aspiration. Overweight and obese people can be seen in every socio-economic group but, in general and at least among women, they are more common in the more deprived communities.

Data from the Oxford-based National Obesity Observatory (NOO) showed that in 2012, 42 per cent of men in England were overweight and nearly 25 per cent were obese. Women were less likely to be overweight (32 per cent) but the same proportion, 25 per cent, were obese. Only a very small proportion – fewer than 2 per cent of adults – were underweight. In women, there is a direct correlation between living in poor circumstances and obesity – 31.5 per cent of those living in the most deprived areas of the country were obese, compared to 21.5 per cent of the least deprived. But there is not the same huge gap for men.[3]

Experts juggle with the inconsistencies in the pattern. There are even more stark differences between the sexes when they are broken down by ethnicity. The highest obesity levels of all are among black African women, more than a third of whom – 38 per cent – were obese in 2004, the latest year in which the data has been collected. But black African men had half that rate: only 17 per cent were obese. The lowest obesity rates were in Bangladeshi and Chinese men (6 per cent) and Chinese women (8 per cent).

People who have had a good education and career are less likely to be overweight – although some people believe there is a discriminatory effect causing fatter people to be less likely to do so well at school and much less likely to be promoted at work. Those with the least education are the most likely to be obese – 29.8 per cent of men and 33 per cent of women who left school without a qualification. The National Obesity Observatory data shows that there are geographic concentrations of high obesity, such as the north-east and the Midlands, where Gateshead and Tamworth respectively tied for the dubious distinction of the fattest towns in England in 2011.

Obesity took off in the 80s, during the 'have it all' Thatcher revolution, when we were told we could be anything we wanted to be if we were bold and determined enough. We should get on our bikes and look for jobs if we were unlucky enough to live in areas of high unemployment. We should pull ourselves up by our bootstraps. It was all down to us. Needless to say, we could eat what we liked and as much as we liked too. Thatcher was delighted by McDonald's, which moved its headquarters into her constituency in 1982, next door to East Finchley underground station. She opened the building in 1983 and visited again on the anniversary of her decade as prime minister in 1989, when she unveiled a plaque on a new extension building. According to the local paper, the *Finchley Times*, she congratulated McDonald's vice-president Paul Preston for employing so many people. Obesity was way off her radar, even though the statistics were showing an alarming rise. This was about the economy, as always. 'You have aimed for higher and higher standards, offer value-for-money food, and added to that you make a profit,' she told Preston.

Neither then nor since has any government been willing to defend those identified by Foresight as vulnerable from the rapacious profiteering of the multinational food manufacturers who produce high-calorie food and sugary drinks or the supermarkets who promote them or the fast-food restaurants that offer cheap deals.

There has been no comprehensive plan from any political party to tackle the obesogenic environment. The unwillingness of we, the public, to talk about fatness, overweight, obesity – call it what you will – allows the politicians to avoid the issues or offer half-hearted responses. Above all else, it enables them to avoid what they fear would be a damaging confrontation with the powerful economic players within the food and drink industry which provide the junk that is doing us harm. Politicians are also afraid they will be accused of taxing the poor if they hike the prices of cheap foods – an argument often put forward by their industry friends. One government after another, since the Foresight report came out, has opted for talks and voluntary agreements on food labelling and marketing to children. The deals that have been struck have been partial and ineffective.

Tony Blair made it clear where he stood in 2004, following a report from the health select committee of the House of Commons which pointed out that Britain had the fastest growing obesity problem in Europe and criticised ministers for not doing enough. On BBC television's *Breakfast with Frost* show, the then Labour prime minister said: 'I am responsible for many things. But I can't make people slimmer.'

By 2006, his rhetoric had changed. He no longer pushed the issue away as one solely for the individual. He had seen how big a bill the country was running up. In a keynote speech on healthy living, the year before he handed the premiership to Gordon Brown, he warned of the cost of doing nothing, describing the obesity epidemic in powerful terms: 'It is worth pausing for a moment to consider the consequences that inaction will bring. The economic burden of chronic disease, including lost work, the early drawing down of pension entitlements and the need for palliative care, could be vast. Heart disease alone costs the UK nearly £8 billion per annum. The health select committee estimate that the full costs of obesity and overweight people to the country is in the region of £7 billion per year.'

He admitted his views had changed. He could now see this was an area where the government should get involved. 'The truth is we all pay a collective price for the failure to take shared responsibility … Now, and particularly where children are concerned, I have come to the conclusion we need to be tougher, more active in setting standards and enforcing them.'

Blair announced bans on fizzy drinks and sweets and crisps in schools. Junk-filled vending machines must go, he said. But when it came to advertising to children, he was not willing to go beyond a voluntary code for industry.

Of course, there would be legislation if the ads did not cease, Blair said. That is a threat all governments have used since, but it has never gone beyond rhetoric.

Governments of every colour want to work hand in hand with those very food manufacturers and fast food chains who need, to be profitable, to keep people buying more and more of their unhealthy food and entice more children, their customers of the future, to want it. As Terence Stephenson, paediatrician and president of the Academy of Medical Royal Colleges put it in 2013, that is like 'putting Dracula in charge of the blood bank'.

Labour's Big Idea came in bright colours and with cartoon characters. Aardman Animations, creators of Wallace and Gromit, were commissioned to produce films to persuade people to eat better and get more physically active. The social marketing campaign was called Change4Life. Labour invested £250 million in it over three years in 2009. Leisure centres and supermarkets were encouraged to use the logo on healthy promotions, such as free swims and money off fruit and vegetables. Asda, Tesco, Unilever, PepsiCo and Kellogg's were among the big food companies supporting the campaign and using the logo. It was a perfect fit with the New Labour government philosophy. It was about working with industry, not against it.

But this was a light-touch approach, hardly the full-frontal assault that is needed. Governments have not always soft-pedalled on health messages. Compare it with the messaging two decades earlier, in 1986, under one of the most right-wing governments Britain has ever elected. Margaret Thatcher's health secretary Norman Fowler also embarked on a national TV advertising campaign against a threat to the nation's health: AIDS. The Don't Die of Ignorance campaign was everything Change4Life was not. It was hard-hitting, scary and effective. The message of the tombstone and the mostly submerged iceberg is remembered by those who saw it even now. AIDS could kill the unsuspecting and unprepared. The impact on unprotected casual sex was marked. The adverts had a major, long-lasting impact – only Sweden, Norway and Finland, which all also mounted hard-hitting AIDS warning campaigns, now have lower HIV levels than the UK in western Europe.[4] Compare this to obesity, where the UK has the worst problem in western Europe.

Obesity is not AIDS, which was killing young people and for which there is no cure. But it is taking a massive toll on health and life, and is responsible for years of misery and disability from diabetes and heart disease. Even if you argue that adults are responsible for their size, children are not. The AIDS campaign proved that people can be shocked into changing their behaviour. Change4Life's jolly little family of blob-like faceless people are likely to evoke nothing more than a rueful smile or more likely a yawn and a flick of the wrist to change TV channels. Governments know this. They have been willing to support more and more graphic images to horrify us out of smoking. Adverts which showed tumours growing out the end of cigarettes attracted numerous complaints to the Advertising Standards Authority, but the government stood firm, insisted it was justified and won its case. The ASA said it understood the ads would have been unsettling, but 'the important health message was justified and the hard-hitting imagery in the ads was suitable given the serious nature of the issue being addressed'.

Where, then, are the ads linking too many soft drinks, burgers and chips to furred-up arteries, cancer and diabetic foot amputations? Either the politicians are running scared of the food industry or they just don't care about the vulnerable, many of them from lower socio-economic classes, who are more likely to pile on weight.

Labour did not do enough. The Conservative/Liberal coalition has been no different. A month before 15-year-old Georgia made the front page of the *Sun*, David Cameron, leader of the Conservative party in opposition, made a key political speech at the start of a by-election campaign in

Glasgow East – an area every bit as economically blighted as south Wales. He knew his words would make no difference to the result; this was a safe Labour seat. But it gave him the opportunity to put down a marker. The problem in communities like this one, he said, is that we have been willing to ascribe a whole range of social ills, from knife violence to poor school results, unemployment and drunkenness, to the deprived environment. We need, said Cameron in July 2008, to end this 'moral neutrality' and talk about good and evil, right and wrong. Cameron was setting out the Tory philosophy on social issues of personal responsibility: so it is your own fault if you are overweight.

'Refusing to use these words – right and wrong – means a denial of personal responsibility and the concept of a moral choice,' he said.[5] We should have the moral fibre to take the right course for ourselves and don't need or want a nanny state telling us what to do. He did take on board what by then had become accepted wisdom – that the salt-and saturated fat-laden food available in takeaways and supermarkets has to change because you can't make healthy choices if the right food is not available at a price you can afford. But his idea of what needed to be done fell a long way short of Foresight's analysis.

Three years later, like Blair before him, it looked as though Cameron was about to have a road to Damascus moment. In 2011, Cameron was reported to be considering the possibility of a 'fat tax'. Denmark had imposed one on food containing more than 2.3 per cent saturated fat. 'The problem in the past when people have looked at using the tax system in this way is the impact it can have on people on low incomes. But frankly, do we have a problem with the growing level of obesity? Yes,' he said.

Nothing further happened.

In 2013, five years after Cameron's Glasgow lecture to poor families on stiffening their moral backbone, Anna Soubry, the government's newly appointed public health minister, also expressed the view that obesity was effectively an issue mainly for the feckless poor. Soubry was a straight-talking, often outspoken minister who probably did want the food and drink industry to move further and faster than it was doing. Her speech on obesity to the Food and Drink Federation in January 2013 echoed David Cameron's views that families must take responsibility for what they and their children eat but it also pointedly urged the food industry to cut more fat and salt from their products. As Labour had before her, she threatened the industry with regulation if they did not move faster.

But her words provoked a furore, because of the clear implication that she saw the obese as part of a hopeless and impoverished underclass. The children of the poor used to be the 'skinny runts' who did not get enough to eat when she was at school, she said. Now they are fat because they get too much. And she squarely blamed their families.

'When I go to my constituency, in fact when I walk around, you can almost now tell somebody's background by their weight,' she said. 'Obviously, not everybody who is overweight comes from deprived backgrounds but that's where the propensity lies.

'It is a heartbreaking fact that people who are some of the most deprived in our society are living on an inadequate diet. But this time it's an abundance of bad food.'

On her way to work at Westminster, she sees parents buying what she called unhealthy 'breakfast buns' for their children, she said. 'They are not rich people, [yet they are] taking their children to school and they buy them breakfast.'

In many homes, it is no longer routine to get up early and eat breakfast together in the morning. 'Where I am in Nottingham, there is a Sainsbury's and you see children going in there buying takeaway food – a sandwich, but more likely a packet of crisps, a fizzy drink – and that's their breakfast.'

She elaborated on the breakdown of family life in poor homes to a journalist from the *Telegraph* who was at the meeting. 'What they don't do is actually sit down and share a meal around the table. There are houses where they don't any longer have dining tables. They will sit in front of the telly and eat,' she said.

'It doesn't mean to say you can't ever sit in front of the telly and have a meal. But I believe children need structure in their lives, they need routine.'

Soubry's observations on the changes in society will be recognised by many and she has a point. Breakfast is often taken on the run, or picked up on the way to work or school by adults and children alike. Dinner, particularly in the week, has to fit around the times that children and parents get home and what there may be in the fridge or freezer depending on whether anyone has had a chance to shop –

as well as the timings of favourite television programmes. Both parents at work, if they can get work, is today's norm.

Soubry was reflecting a state of affairs that is very familiar to many of us – but her words were taken as a damning assumption that this only happens in poor households. Above all, she was attacked for her condescending tone. Her words were taken to imply that the obese are not like us. That may have been what she meant, though later she denied it. What was for certain was that her attempt to start a discussion about the reality of obesity in our lives was rejected by newspapers, which gunned for the messenger and rejected the message.

A few months later in a debate in the House of Commons on childhood obesity and diabetes, Soubry argued she had been misrepresented and claimed some 'political cheap shots' had been aimed at her. She also made an extraordinary and fascinating comment which was not picked up, but amounted to a damning indictment of the governing classes. 'Obesity, as everyone attending this debate knows, is effectively a killer,' she said. 'If we were absolutely honest about it, if obesity were a disease, governments of whatever political colour would have taken action many, many years ago to tackle the growing problem – no pun intended – of obesity and being overweight, notably in our children.'

That was quite an admission from a minister for public health. Soubry was admitting that governments have neglected obesity – as they still do.

You get the feeling that, deep down, Soubry really did care about the overweight, but was constrained by her position as part of a pro-business government which was determined to fly the flag of personal responsibility. It was not the only issue in public health where she seemed at odds with some of her Cabinet colleagues. Perhaps this underlying tension – and what was described as her tendency to shoot from the hip – was responsible for her transfer from health to defence in the reshuffle of October 2013. The interview that I had sought with her to discuss her views – which she appeared to have been avoiding – was finally off the agenda.

While in her post, Soubry toed the party line. Like Cameron, she made no concession to the obesogenic environment that had been identified in the Foresight report as the real problem. She was not inclined to blame the food industry in public. So it was the overweight themselves who were held responsible, a disproportionate number of whom were from deprived communities as a result of the vulnerability that Foresight talks about. But telling them to be tougher about resisting the unhealthy offerings of the food manufacturers at the very least lacks understanding of the situation. Fast, cheap and convenient meals and snacks are specifically targeted at those people who are short of money as well as time.

Indeed, food manufacturers spend billions on marketing their unhealthy but filling junk. In 2010, the Yale Rudd Center for food policy and obesity reported that fast-food companies such as Burger King and Pizza Hut spent $4 billion marketing their often high-fat, high-salt wares in the US, attracting clever and imaginative minds to work on their campaigns. It is not a fair fight.

'Individuals exist within a social environment,' said Simon Capewell, professor of public health and policy at Liverpool University. 'Certainly government would like to say it is all down to the individual and everybody has free choice. This is moderate nonsense. They don't have the education, the money and health literacy, peer support or examples. They are literally drowning in a sea of marketing messages.

'The government was spending £75 million a year on Change4Life, now cut to £14 million. The food and drink industry spend over £1 billion a year on marketing in the UK.'

In May 2010, the coalition government formed by the Tories and Liberal Democrats came to power. The coalition quickly stopped all funding of social marketing programmes, including Change4Life, pending an assessment of their impact and a decision on whether they were worth the money (a year later, it resumed support of Change4Life at a much reduced level). Instead, the coalition's Big Idea on tackling obesity was the Responsibility Deal.

Andrew Lansley, while still shadow health secretary, set up a public health commission in August 2009 to look at the idea of a deal between government, business and 'the third sector', including health groups, in which the food industry would agree to voluntary health improvements to its products and restraints on marketing to children. Industry was at the table from the outset. It was chaired by Dave Lewis, who was also chairman of Unilever UK and Ireland, manufacturers of margarine, mayonnaise and ice creams.

The deal became a reality and the flagship Tory public health strategy early in 2011. Manufacturers, takeaway

restaurant chains and supermarket groups sat around
the table with health organisations and agreed to pledge
voluntary reductions in the amount of salt and fat in their
products – and eventually calories too. But the process
was slow, only included those companies that chose to
get involved and it was hard to ascertain what the changes
really meant.

Critics of the deal included an independent expert
group which had been set up to advise government on
obesity in line with a recommendation of the Foresight
report by Labour. The committee quickly became a thorn
in the coalition government's side, suggesting that tackling
obesity was far more complex than Lansley's initiatives
presupposed. It did not have much time for 'nudge' – the
Tory philosophy adapted from the book by Thaler and
Sunstein that you can bring about behaviour change by
hints and suggestions of the right path to follow, rather
than intervening with heavy-handed legislation.

Before long, the advisory committee members went
public with their concerns. Geof Rayner and Tim Lang
wrote a piece for the *British Medical Journal* attacking the
plausibility of 'nudge'. In April 2011, Rayner and Lang
wrote that obesity was by now recognised to be the result
of the 'complex multifactorial interplay' of over-eating,
reduced physical activity, food oversupply, marketing,
pricing, poor consumer choice, genetics and many other
things. 'So why is the British government quietly breaking
with this consensus and putting so much weight behind
nudge thinking?' they asked.

'Although the last government started the drift into this thinking via Change4Life as a social marketing approach, the coalition government has narrowed the strategy further,' wrote Rayner and Lang. In what may have been their committee's death knell, they concluded with their fear 'that nudge becomes collusion between the state and corporations to hoodwink consumers. At least nannies are overt.'

In November 2011, the committee was disbanded. The government announced that it was making different advisory arrangements and dismissed the group, holding onto only Susan Jebb of the Medical Research Council, who chaired both it and the food Responsibility Deal committee.

Professor Klim McPherson of Oxford University, who was on the Foresight review and the subsequent advisory committee, said their criticisms of the government's policy had led to their disbanding. 'Too many of us were giving critical voice to the Responsibility Deal and its effectiveness,' he told me at the time. The advisory committee members wanted a far more aggressive government policy to stem the rise in obesity, including interventions industry did not want, such as fat taxes and proper labelling, 'which government wasn't going to do'.

'They ignored us,' he said. 'Then rather than ignoring us, they disbanded us. Government policy is not concerned with what central government can do – it is more concerned with what industry can do.'

Rayner, honorary research fellow at City University in London, believes the blame games that governments play are very wrong. 'What we're talking about is a lot of communities having very poor diets, completely unable to afford a better one,' he said. 'They are having processed food as the norm. I find it so objectionable that the poorest people are being told it is their fault.'

One month before the advisory committee was disbanded, in October 2011, health secretary Andrew Lansley announced an obesity Call to Action to slash five billion calories from the national diet – the equivalent, said his department helpfully, of 16.9 million cheeseburgers, which would cover 20 football pitches, or 28,409,091 caffe lattes, which would fill four Olympic swimming pools.

Lansley called on the food companies to cut the calorie content of the products they make by about 3–5 per cent, which would result in the entire population losing weight without even thinking about it. It sounded like one of those miracle diets that invites you to slim while you sleep. It was greeted with ridicule.

'This whole strategy is just worthless, regurgitated, patronising rubbish,' said Jamie Oliver, the TV chef turned food campaigner. 'Any of us could walk into any primary school in the country and find plenty of eight-year-olds with more creative solutions to these problems. It's a farce.' He called for the government to make real change and then legislate and finance it.

Usually less vocal critics also poured scorn on the proposal. Terence Stephenson, president of the Royal College of Paediatrics and Child Health, said the five billion calorie target 'may grab headlines but is actually peanuts – 16 dry-roasted peanuts per person, per day, to be precise'.

He said: 'The plan has no clear measures on how the food and drink industry will be made to be more responsible in their aggressive marketing of unhealthy food.'

Richard Lloyd, executive director of the consumer magazine *Which?* said the government was being naïve about the food industry. 'Food and drink manufacturers must cut fat and sugar, and therefore calories, from their products where possible and promote healthier options. But expecting them to do this voluntarily through a vague call to action is naïve. We need a proper strategy which includes ambitious targets,' he said.

Although the Call to Action was aimed at the food and drink industry, Lansley was not departing from Cameron's script that we as individuals all have to take responsibility. Lest we should think that, Dame Sally Davis, chief medical officer, was also at the launch to do a little light hectoring of the population (heaven forbid anyone should call it nannying). 'We all have a role to play, from businesses to local authorities, but as individuals we all need to take responsibility. This means thinking about what we eat and thinking about the number of calories in our diets to maintain a healthy weight,' she said.

And Professor Alan Jackson of SACN (the government's scientific advisory committee on nutrition) was there to provide scientific back-up. We might be surprised to find out that we are all consuming about 10 per cent more calories than we need, he said. Unfortunately, just to confuse the message, the committee had decided that the number of calories we all need for a healthy life is actually higher

– not lower – than previous estimates. A man needs an average of 2605 calories a day and a woman needs 2079, which is around 100 extra calories than had previously been thought. But, of course, said the panel quickly, we are all exceeding that. An obese man eats an average of 500 calories a day more than a man of normal weight. And so the numbers were tossed to and fro. More confusion, less enlightenment and no progress.

From 2011 onwards, the nation's weight problems slipped almost entirely off the government agenda as the perpetual recession kept attention focused on the economy and on jobs. Public health became the responsibility of local government, placing a huge burden on the authorities in south Wales, in the Midlands, in the north-east and in other regions where obesity rates are far higher than in Westminster. These areas will pay a price in ill-health much earlier than in the affluent south of England.

There have been few changes to the environment where Georgia Davis grew up that facilitate healthy living. Aberdare has a covered market near the station, where plenty of fruit and vegetables and meat and fish are for sale, alongside knitting wool and clothes and gimmicks and gadgets. But the main shopping streets of the town offer every kind of cheap takeaway, from pizzas to pies to chips to curry. The Pop-In Cafe will do you home-made chicken curry, with both rice and chips – as well as a free can of fizzy drink, tea or coffee – for £4.60. A Wetherspoon pub appears to be the most upmarket dining option, and has the calories on the menu – the big chain signed up to the government's Responsibility Deal. A handful of dishes are advertised as coming in at under 500 calories, but that's not what most people are eating. Fish and chips, at 1258 calories, is a more popular choice.

To reach the housing estate where Georgia was brought up, you have to climb a steep road out of the shopping streets that runs up the far side of the valley. A lot of cars are passing, where once adults and children would have had no option but to walk. There is nobody on the pavement, but it is a wet day.

On the right-hand side of the road is a general store, closed and boarded. The glass door is shattered and a wooden panel has been nailed over it. On the ground by the step is a crushed cola can. Facing the traffic heading up the hill is a large billboard. 'Tuck in at Night', says the advert. It is for McDonald's, which has, it says, over 500 restaurants open 24 hours a day. It invites you to download the McDonald's app to find your closest all-night eatery.

Georgia is not in the yellowish-cream semi-detached house, one of many identical homes on the estate. The shape of the hole made in the upstairs outside wall is still faintly visible under new brickwork and a coat of paint. Her mother appears at the door. 'She doesn't live here any more,' she said. 'But she won't speak to you. She has a contract with the *Sun*.'

Nobody wants to talk about obesity, unless there are lurid details and there's money to be made. It's not about us anyway. We are all in denial.

2

SUGAR, FAT AND ALCOHOL: A DEADLY TRIO

Rivers of Coca-Cola, torrents of Fanta and waterfalls of Dr Pepper bubble through the bottling process at a plant on the edge of the North Circular Road around London at a rate of up to 142,000 litres an hour. The factory in Edmonton is not quite Willy Wonka's fantastical children's paradise, but its production capacity is mind-blowing. It is short on Oompa Loompas, but it has machines that can blow plastic bottles into shape and fill them at the same time. And there is another link to Roald Dahl's fictional Chocolate Factory – the drinks produced here are up to one-third sugar.

White gold, sugar was once called, because it was so profitable. A number of very vocal experts now think this precious commodity could be damaging our health. Some say it is the main reason we are increasingly overweight and obese. But sugar is deeply embedded not only in our eating and drinking habits but is also a fundamental and important part of the world economy. The governments of countries that produce it, including the USA and the UK, are fiercely protective. They are not about to damage sales.

The importance of sugar and the products that use large quantities of it to the UK was clear when the industry won a battle for the abolition of quotas in the European Union in June 2013. It was to Coca-Cola in Edmonton that the government minister for food and farming, David Heath, headed for a celebratory visit – not to a cake, biscuit or sweet factory. The British Soft Drinks Association took him there. That tells us two things. Firstly, it reminds us of the huge importance of sugar to the soft drinks industry. A standard can of Coca-Cola contains 35g of sugar: that is nearly nine teaspoons of sugar, which is marginally more than in a Mars bar.[1] And secondly, it tells us that the soft drinks industry is big, profitable and matters to the British economy. Heath said during the visit: 'EU sugar quotas, which are driving up the wholesale price of sugar by as much as 35 per cent, are a prime example of the kind of barriers to growth that government is working hard to remove. I came here not only to see a leading company committed to improving both efficiency and sustainability, but also to find out what more government can do to help Britain's food and drink industry grow economically and compete in the global race.'

The British government, in other words, just as in the US and other sugar-producing countries, has a vested interest in the sweet stuff.

Coca-Cola and other sugar-laden soft drinks are toxic, some health campaigners believe. They have been indicted as a prime cause of the obesity epidemic. But health ministers around the world are keeping pretty quiet on the subject. It is the food and farming ministers and the Treasury who call the shots. Because of the profits and the taxes from soft drinks and processed foods and the numbers of people the industry employs, governments will sit on their hands unless forced to act.

The noise over sugar has been growing, but ministers turn a deaf ear. It is your choice to drink sugary Coke, they say. Diet Coke and Zero are available for anybody who is watching their weight, adds the multinational corporation, which sponsored the Olympics to plant associations in our minds between fitness and fizzy drinks. There is no good scientific evidence that sugar causes obesity, say industry lobbyists, and besides, sugar consumption has dropped slightly over the past decade, while obesity has gone up by 15 per cent.

This last may be true – although the figures are, as always, based on highly questionable dietary surveys. When researchers ask how often people eat fattening foods or consume sugary drinks, some of us feel unaccountably guilty and lie, while others just can't remember. So sugar may not be the only reason we have got fat, but it certainly looks like one of them.

What has changed radically is the way we eat sugar. We used to buy it in bags or boxes of glittering cubes and set it out in china bowls on the tea table where children like me stole lumps to crunch surreptitiously in corners. We baked it into our cakes and puddings. But that household use of sugar has slumped dramatically over the last 40 years, to be almost completely replaced by hidden sugars. You can't see most of the sugar you now eat.

There is sugar in bread – around 1.5g in a slice, which is more than a third of a teaspoon. There is sugar in breakfast cereals, where you might expect it, and in salad dressing and pizza and savoury ready meals where you might not. There are more than five teaspoons or cubes of sugar in 100g of ketchup or nearly a whole cube in a single 17g serving. A supermarket-bought 250g Margherita pizza made by Pizza Express contains nearly 3 cubes of sugar. It is supposedly intended for two, so a couple sharing would be eating one and a half cubes of sugar each in what they would have thought was a savoury dinner. But many people would eat a whole one on their own.

What we do know is that our consumption of all those deceptively sugar-rich processed foods has climbed dramatically. According to IASO, the International Association for the Study of Obesity, we were buying 535g of sugar per person per week for household use in 1974 and consuming 267g in processed food and drinks and meals out.[2] By 2007, that balance was inverted, to 125g for home use and 568g of sugar in our bought food. We no longer add sugar to what we eat – but the food industry does.

Our liking for sweetness is as old as mankind, says Walter Willett, Fredrick John Stare professor of epidemiology and nutrition at the Harvard School of Public Health. 'We clearly have sweetness receptors. We are genetically programmed to seek out sweet foods. Where did that come from? The taste for sweetness was to detect tender young leaves with some sources of energy. It was evolutionarily very important,' he said.

'But we have taken the sense of sweetness and ratcheted it up in quite an enormous way. That is getting us into trouble. The food industry has massively tried to exploit that sensation.'

Sugar is as dangerous as controlled drugs, says Robert Lustig, the US paediatrician who turned campaigner against sugar after treating too many desperately overweight children. He says there are at least 40 different names for the hidden sugar in our food, such as maltose and dextran, making it hard to spot on the label and harder to control what he believes is our addiction. As with cigarettes, we're in the grip of a habit we can't easily kick.

'We need to wean ourselves off. We need to de-sweeten our lives, we need to make sugar a treat, not a diet staple,' he told me on a visit to London to talk about his book *Fat Chance: The Bitter Truth About Sugar*. 'The food industry has currently made it into a diet staple because they know when they do, you buy more. This is their hook. If some unscrupulous cereal manufacturer went out and laced your breakfast cereal with morphine to get you to buy more, what would you think of that? They do it with sugar instead.'

The addiction theory is growing in currency. The work of Nora Volkow, director of the National Institute on Drug Abuse in the United States, is central. She and colleagues moved from studying the effects of cocaine on the brain, to what happens when some of us eat fatty foods or drink sweetened colas. They found that there are similar dopamine surges in the brain, fuelling a desire for drugs or for sugar. It is controversial, and she is the first to say so, because nobody is addicted to food in the same way that they are to crack cocaine. But if Volkow, great-granddaughter of Leon Trotsky, is right, her work will have repercussions around the world and perhaps particular significance in Mexico, land of her birth, which has the highest Coca-Cola consumption in the world.[3]

Sugar has an exotic history, which made slaves of some men and brought vast wealth to others. In Silvertown in London's docklands still stands the largest cane sugar refinery in Europe, built by Henry Tate in 1878, whose business was later merged with that of Abram Lyle, producer of golden syrup. Overlooking the Thames nine miles upriver is the Tate Gallery, built in all its marble elegance with sugar money to house some of the world's finest paintings, starting with Tate's own pre-Raphaelite collection. Between them now is the Tate Modern, in a converted power station on the South Bank, which lends the contrast of its Victorian industrial grandeur to the 21st century art it contains.

Tate and Lyle's products are made from imported cane sugar, once from the colonies in the Americas. The enormous profits to be made triggered the trade in slaves from Africa to work on the plantations and played a crucial role in helping Britain become one of the world's greatest powers in the 17th and 18th centuries.

Sugar has always been an industry with its roots deep in the British establishment. Sugar beet began to be grown in Norfolk in the early 20th century. By 1936, the 18 sugar-beet factories that had sprung up around the country were amalgamated as British Sugar and until 1981 the British government remained a shareholder. British Sugar is still the sole company processing sugar beet, but now, as is the way of the modern world, it is part of the massive conglomerate known as Associated British Foods, which also owns Twinings tea, Ovaltine, Jordans Ryvita and the blockbuster of all retailers, Primark.

In the UK and many other countries, Coca-Cola is sweetened with sugar. The USA uses high fructose corn syrup – now frequently abbreviated to HFCS – which became cheap because of agricultural over-production and farming subsidies from government. In 2004, HFCS began to be blamed in the US for the obesity epidemic, following a groundbreaking paper from the US experts George Bray and Barry Popkin, which pointed out that the steady rise in the use of corn syrup matched the upward obesity trajectory. That allowed the sugar manufacturers to claim they were off the hook. HFCS instead was in the frame.

Sugar wars broke out. As concern rose in the United States, the corn syrup manufacturers fought back, first launching a multimillion-dollar advertising campaign saying HFCS was no different from sugar, and then in 2010 petitioning the Food and Drink Authority to change the name corn syrup to corn sugar – similar to cane sugar. The US Sugar Association promptly filed a lawsuit against the Corn Refiners Association for false advertising, insisting HFCS and sugar are fundamentally different.

But, say Popkin and Bray today, the demonisation of high fructose corn syrup ignores the central point. The problem is fructose in whatever form. And they both contain the substance in high quantities: sugar is 50 per cent fructose and HFCS is 55 per cent fructose (although sometimes more).

'The concern with HFCS in our diet has led to a reduced proportion of HFCS in beverages compared to other sugars,' the pair wrote in a study updating their work in the journal *Paediatric Obesity* in 2013. 'This paper shows that this is a misplaced shift.' They show that drinks which now have reduced high fructose corn syrup, and are now advertised as better for you because of it, simply have other sugars as a substitute, which still contain at least 50 per cent fructose. Heads you lose, tails you lose.

Of course, many people in the USA and Europe are switching to diet drinks and bottled water, as concern over sugar mounts. But Popkin, from the University of North Carolina at Chapel Hill School of Public Health, is now worried about the increase in drinks that appear to be harmless because they are natural. What could be more healthy than fruit? But fruit juice and smoothies contain large amounts of fructose, because they are made by extracting the juice from many fruits, not just one.

'Smoothies and fruit juice are the new danger,' Popkin told me. 'It's kind of the next step in the evolution of the battle. And it's a really big part of it because in every country they've been replacing soft drinks with fruit juice and smoothies as the new healthy beverage. So you will find that Coke and Pepsi have bought dozens [of fruit juice companies] around the globe.'

So they have. In the UK, Coca-Cola bought Innocent Smoothies, a brand with a squeaky clean image. PepsiCo bought Tropicana. Launching Tropicana Smoothies in 2008, PepsiCo's sales pitch was that the drink would help the nation to reach its 'five a day' fruit and vegetable target. 'Smoothies are one of the easiest ways to boost daily fruit intake as each 250ml portion contains the equivalent of two fruit portions,' it said.

But the five a day advice needs to change, says Popkin. Vegetable juice is fine. Fruit juice, stripped of its fibre and in the quantity of fruits required to make a single drink, is not. 'Think of eating one orange or two and getting filled,' he said. 'Now think of drinking a smoothie with six oranges and two hours later it does not affect how much you eat. The entire literature shows that we feel full from drinking beverages like smoothies but it does not affect our overall food intake, whereas eating an orange does. So pulped-up smoothies do nothing good for us but do give us the same amount of sugar as four to six oranges or a large Coke. It is deceiving.'

In pursuit of a healthy sweetener, food and drink companies are turning in droves to fruit juice concentrates, he says. Look at the 'natural sweetener' on the labelling of health-food snacks and drinks. It may well be fruit juice – high in fructose. 'The most important issue about added sugar is that everybody thinks it's cane sugar or maybe beet sugar or HFC syrup or all the other syrups but globally the cheapest thing on the market almost is fruit juice concentrate coming out of China,' said Popkin. 'It has created an overwhelming supply of apple juice concentrate. It is being used everywhere and it also gets around the sugar quotas that lots of countries have.'

He and some colleagues did a survey of sweeteners in 600,000 US food products between 2005 and 2009 for a paper published in 2012. They found that fruit juice concentrate was the fifth most common sweetener overall and the second most common, after HFCS, in soft drinks – and also in babies' formula milk.

He admits that there are not yet the solid, long-term studies that are needed to prove that fruit juice is the issue he fears. There are only two really good long-term trials – one in Singapore and one by Harvard, he says. 'But all the long-term studies on fruit juice in anything show the same kind of effect whether it's a smoothie or natural [juice] and whether it's a diabetes or weight-gain effect,' he said.

And we are consuming more and more of the stuff. Spread across the population, we each drank the equivalent of 17.6 litres of 'no added sugar' fruit juice and smoothies in 2012. The fructose content of these drinks is huge. Orange juice typically contains the equivalent of five cubes of sugar in a 250ml serving – that's as much as four chocolate digestive biscuits. An Innocent strawberry and banana smoothie has more than six – about the same as a Crunchie bar. So we are consuming the equivalent of around 350 cubes of sugar a year each, thanks solely to our 'healthy' fruit juice habit.

That doesn't let sugar-sweetened fizzy drinks off the hook. Most obesity experts are still focused on the dangers of colas and lemonades and other soft drinks with added sugar or HFCS, because of the sheer quantity we drink. The resultant growing public alarm has registered with the manufacturers, who now are quick to point out that sales of the diet versions and bottled waters they make are rising.[4]

The biggest problem with all soft drinks – and the reason why global concern is so much focused on Coke rather than cookies or chocolate – is that they do not fill you up. Most people can drink sugary drinks without affecting their appetite for more food. 'If you take a candy bar you cut the calories in something else you eat,' said Popkin. Fanta or Sprite do not make you feel satiated. You eat everything else you would have eaten as well.

So cutting our sugar intake from soft drinks look like an easier win than reforming our entire diet. That's why Mayor Bloomberg in New York has fought to ban super-sized cups of soda from restaurants and why British health campaigners are calling for a soft drinks tax in the UK. In January 2013, Sustain published its 'Children's Future Fund' report, urging that £1 billion a year could be raised from a tax of 20p a litre and invested in children's health programmes. It has been backed by over 60 organisations and supported by the former children's commissioner, Al Aynsley-Green. The following month, the Academy of Medical Royal Colleges also called for the tax.

But the soft drinks companies' efforts to grow the market continue unabashed. Coca-Cola in the UK declared its ambition in 2013 to increase the UK market by £2.1 billion by 2017, identifying six 'moments' in the day when we could be persuaded to buy more soft drinks, including fruit juice and smoothies for breakfast and soft drinks for children when they come home from school. Sales of Coca-Cola still outstrip those of Diet Coke and Zero Coke combined. The company continues to insist it is up to us – if we are worried about our weight, we should look at everything we eat and drink, instead of picking on them.

'We believe that rather than single out any ingredient, it is more helpful for people to look at their total energy balance,' said Coca-Cola in a statement.

You can argue that people should know better than to consume vast quantities of sugary drinks, but that is to pretend we do not live in a world where it is cheap, easy and normal to do so. Lunchtime for many people at work in shops and offices is about a 'meal deal'. A sandwich, a cake or crisps and a drink come as a bargain package. There is a choice of drinks, but young people I have talked to say they don't feel they are getting value if they choose water, which they could get from a tap, so they choose Coke or Pepsi in a bottle with a screw top, that they can finish later at their desk. It's convenient.

Coca-Cola, PepsiCo and other companies spend billions on marketing, urging us to drink more. One of the claims they are increasingly making is that we need to rehydrate. Never mind that we would best be doing that with water. Amid the noisy selling of fun and pleasure, we don't hear the real health message, which is to lay off the sugar.

In 2003, the World Health Organisation tried to increase the volume. In a draft report entitled *Diet, Nutrition and the Prevention of Chronic Disease*, it proposed that sugar should not account for more than 10 per cent of anybody's calorie intake, on the grounds of potential damage to teeth as well as the risk of obesity.

The reaction was immediate and hostile. The sugar lobby brought out the big guns. The Sugar Association in the United States wrote to Gro Harlem Brundtland, the director general of the World Health Organisation, threatening to use its considerable influence in Congress to block US funding. In the letter, it said it would 'exercise every avenue available to expose the dubious nature' of the WHO's report on diet and nutrition, including challenging its $406m (£260m) funding from the US. It insisted the science on which the 10 per cent limit was based was flawed – and that sugar, just another form of carbohydrate, could safely account for 25 per cent of a healthy diet.

'Taxpayers' dollars should not be used to support misguided, non-science-based reports which do not add to the health and wellbeing of Americans, much less the rest of the world,' said the letter.

The association, together with six other big food industry groups, also wrote to the US health secretary, Tommy Thompson, asking him to use his influence to get the WHO report withdrawn. The coalition included the US Council for International Business, comprising more than 300 companies – among them Coca-Cola and PepsiCo.

The WHO refused to budge, arguing that a team of 30 independent experts had considered the scientific evidence. Its conclusions were in line with the findings of 23 national reports which had, on average, set targets of 10 per cent for added sugars, it said. The 10 per cent limit stood, but was rubbished and ignored by the sugar lobby and its supporters. There is global confusion as a result. Coca-Cola cans in Mexico are still labelled with a guide-line dietary sugar limit of 25 per cent. The UK government stuck with the advice of its committee on the medical aspects of food policy (COMA) and set a limit of 11 per cent of food energy from what it called 'non-milk extrinsic sugars'.[5] Unlike other countries, that excludes lactose in milk, making the actual UK limit higher than it appears. The NHS Choices website which gives guidance to the public, however, talks of 10 per cent.

What happened in 2003 was a blueprint for every attempt there has been since to discuss limits on sugar consumption – on the grounds of health – on the world stage. Public health experts who are not paid by the industry advise cuts in the amount of sugar we eat. Scientists who take the industry shilling produce research papers disputing their evidence. It is just like the tobacco wars all over again.

Ten years after the stand-off with the US sugar lobby, the WHO's nutrition guidance expert advisory group (NUGAG) dared once more to dip a toe into the shark-filled scientific and political waters. It decided to update the sugar recommendation and commissioned two reviews of the evidence. One was to try to answer the fundamental question everyone is now asking – whether sugar is really a cause of obesity. The other was to assess the damage it does to teeth. A team led by New Zealand-based Professor Jim Mann from the department of human nutrition and medicine of the University of Otago carried out the obesity review and published the results in January 2013 in the *British Medical Journal.*

The paper said that people get fat from eating sugar because they take in too many calories, rather than because of any intrinsic effect of sugar itself on our metabolism. Industry and lobbyists immediately declared sugar itself was exonerated: it's the people who eat too much of it who are to blame. But the Mann review did not leave it there. Sugary food and drinks give you a large number of calories all at once. People rapidly put on weight if they eat a sugar-heavy diet. That means, they said, that advice on cutting down on sugar consumption 'is a relevant component of a strategy to reduce the high risk of overweight and obesity in most countries'. In other words, with a global obesity epidemic raging, it's a pretty good idea for the WHO to tell people they'd be well advised to eat less sugar. In March 2014 the WHO reiterated the 10% limit, but with an ambition to cut sugar to 5% of calories – less than one can of Coke for an average adult.

Mann was more forthright when I spoke to him than he could be in the coded language of a scientific paper. Sugar, he told me, 'unquestionably contributes to obesity', although he thinks some anti-sugar campaigners have gone too far. 'We've got to try to find the happy medium. I don't think sugar is the cause of all evil. It's an important factor and if we're eating more sugar and less fat then we need to take note of it.'

And sugar is not like some other foods in the way it affects our appetite, he said. It is an energy-dense carbohydrate. He told me of a trial where people were instructed to give up sugary foods and eat the same amount of calories from starchy carbohydrates instead – foods like breads and potatoes. They couldn't do it. 'They really didn't like it. They felt full. They weren't complaining about anything to do with addiction – they just felt stuffed with food,' he said.

But here's the biggest problem: although sugary drinks are energy dense, they don't give you that feeling of fullness that stops you wanting more. 'It seems that probably the body doesn't sense calories that come from sugary drinks, so that if one has a Coke with all the vast amount of sugar that it contains you don't register that you've had all these calories,' he said.

It's younger people who are in danger, he thinks, rather than the over-50s, who may well prefer a cup of tea or coffee. 'But if you look for instance at New Zealand, where I am – Pacific youth for example, who are among the fattest people in the world – sugary drinks probably contribute an enormous amount, as indeed in American youth,' he said. In fact, he mused, it is probably the same among young people the whole world over.

For every scientific study that says sugar is a problem, there are half a dozen industry-funded reinterpretations and rebuttals. Big Soda and Big Food fund research and recruit respectable scientists as advisors, just as Big Tobacco did. It's a lot easier with sugar than with cigarettes – nobody was ever able to argue that we needed a puff of nicotine and tar, but we do need food. The heart of the food and drink industry's defence of sugar is that it is just another carbohydrate, and we all need carbohydrates. So there are many scientists who buy the argument that there is nothing wrong with our food – just our attitude to food. It presumably follows that you could get all your carbohydrate needs from toffees and Red Bull.

We, the public, are being misled. We are ill served by many of the bodies that are held up as experts in food and nutrition because they are not impartial. They take money from the big corporations, often with a clear conscience because they don't see any harm in the processed foods and drinks around us. The logic is simple – but those who apply it are blinkered. It's true that a bottle of cola or a kingsize chocolate bar won't kill you. It won't, by itself, have any adverse effect on your health. So a scientist can say with a clear conscience that one snack is as good as another. It's all food. But that totally ignores the big picture – big and getting bigger. We don't eat just one bar or one packet of crisps or one burger a week. We eat junk all the time, in addition to the rest of our meals. Our sugar-load is way above what it should be and so is our saturated fat.

So when the impressively named British Nutrition Foundation publishes a 'facts behind the headlines' paper to debunk Lustig's allegation that sugar is toxic, we need to know a little more about them. The foundation claims independence, but is full of scientists who believe in working with industry and it is funded extensively by the world's largest food corporations. Its 'sustaining members' include Coca-Cola, Danone Waters and Dairies, Dupont, Kellogg, Mondelēz International (spun off from Kraft), Nestlé, PepsiCo, Tate and Lyle, Associated British Foods (which includes British Sugar) and Unilever.

The rebuttal paper said that 'overall, evidence does not support the claims made that sugar increases the risk of diseases like obesity, diabetes and heart disease', but added that 'there is some evidence that high intakes of sugars in the form of sugar-sweetened beverages might contribute to weight gain'.[6] The foundation preferred the views of the European Food Safety Authority (EFSA), which suggested the data on the effects of consuming large amounts of sugar were 'limited and mainly short-term'.[7]

So what about EFSA? This is a body that has itself been embroiled in controversy over conflicts of interest. The chair of its management board, Diana Banati, was censured in 2010 when it was discovered she was also holding a position with the food industry scientific lobbying group International Life Sciences Institute (ILSI). Because of the fuss, she resigned her ILSI post – but in 2012 left EFSA to return to ILSI as its executive and scientific director. Perhaps unsurprisingly, her critics claimed she had been on the food industry's side all along.

And then there is the UK government's very own advisory body. This is SACN, the scientific advisory committee on nutrition. On this important body are a number of scientists who work with big food companies and see nothing wrong with it.

Chairing the SACN working group reviewing carbohydrates in our diet – including and, given the current controversy, especially sugar – is Professor Ian Macdonald from Nottingham University. He is a paid advisor to Coca-Cola and Mars, although he stepped down for the duration of SACN's sugar inquiry. He sees no reason why he should not work for industry. In fact, he thinks it's a good thing. He believes it gives him perspective.

'I have explained my associations with industry to the department of health and they are quite happy with the relationships,' he told me. 'I think it's a more balanced view than some of the views of my nutritional colleagues and also than some of the industrial views. Some of the industrial people can't see what they're doing wrong. That's not right – they do need to start helping people to consume sensible amounts of food and be less sedentary than they are at the moment. But as far as sugar goes, it's difficult to know where to begin because there are people who believe it is the cause of all of our problems. [Professor] John Yudkin started this in the 1970s with *Pure, White and Deadly* and other people have picked it up at intervals beyond. The consumption rates are a bit higher than they were in the 60s, but not excessively so. Consumption hasn't trebled.'

Nonetheless, he has advised Coca-Cola that they have an issue, he said – a perceptual issue. 'I have told the chief executive of Coca-Cola in Atlanta that he has a real problem because his company is perceived as being a cause of the problem and they really do need to do something about their promotion of full-strength Coca-Cola and its status within the business and so on. His senior colleagues winced when I said that to him in the board that I sat on but actually he took it on the chin and they are beginning to do something about it.'

His view is that 'there is a job for industry to do but you get them to do it by talking to them, not by shouting at them and trying to put them out of business'.

That attitude got him recruited to the government's Responsibility Deal with industry, where he is on the calorie reduction expert group. With him sits Professor Judy Buttriss, director general of the British Nutrition Foundation and Dr David Mela from Unilever, who is also a member of the SACN carbohydrate inquiry. Macdonald has become the academic lead for his university's 'strategic relationship' with Unilever, a company that owns ice-cream brands as well as margarine and weight-loss products. Another member of the carbohydrate inquiry has accepted funding from the industry body Sugar Nutrition[8] as well as from the Dairy Council.

In spite of the establishment figures who advise government and try to tell us all that sugar is just fine, there has been a grassroots revolt. We now know that colas are full of sugar – nine spoonfuls a can. We are increasingly aware of the secret sugar in our pizzas and pastas and soups. The trade bodies, Sugar Nutrition in the UK and its global counterpart, the London-based World Sugar Research

Organisation, are increasingly entrenched, yet defiant.[9] Both argue there is no good scientific evidence to blame sugar for obesity. They cite one study after another, most of them industry-funded, on the benefits of sugar. 'No foods should be considered as "good or bad" as all foods play an important role in the diet. It is only when foods are eaten in excess that health problems result,' says the Sugar Nutrition website – exactly the same sort of phrasing used by government ministers and officials.

And they try to deflect the argument onto other food-stuffs. It's not sugar that's the problem – it's fat, says Sugar Nutrition. Well, they would, wouldn't they? 'The balance of available evidence suggests very strongly that eating a diet that contains a high proportion of fat encourages an increase in body-fat stores,' it says, curiously citing a study by Bray and Popkin in 1998, before they published the work on high fructose corn syrup in 2003 that caused all the problems for the soft-drink industry. The other study quoted is by the Danish researcher Arne Astrup in 2001. Astrup, who has a number of citations on the site, is listed in the *American Journal of Clinical Nutrition* 2012 as an advisor to a significant number of food as well as pharmaceutical companies. Sugar Nutrition's website references some studies from the mid-90s that claim lean people eat more sugar than fat people. There is also a study alleging that eating sugar can help people diet. Surprise! It is funded by Sugar Nutrition.

For all their bullish stance, the sugar trade bodies look to be on the back foot. The World Sugar Research Organisation's director general, Richard Cottrell, who was previously director of Sugar Nutrition, no longer seems inclined to share his objective views of the science. 'I don't speak to the press,' he said when I called him – and put the phone down.

While scientists paid by industry abound on other expert bodies, as we have seen, the World Health Organisation is desperate to be seen to be non-partial after various past conflict-of-interest stories. It insists its advisors and committee members like Mann must have no links with industry. Indeed, director general Margaret Chan, in a speech in Helsinki, Finland, in June 2013 on the fight against non-communicable diseases like diabetes and heart conditions and stroke, delivered an indictment of Big Food that stunned her audience. Chan, a Chinese national, had recently secured a second term at the helm of the WHO, which may have made her more willing to speak out, but for any politician, a denunciation of the food corporations would be tricky. Chan has not shown herself to be this bold in the past. She came to the WHO from the Hong Kong government, where, as director of health, she had to deal with the serious global threats first of bird flu and then SARS. She showed herself to be tough in a crisis, ordering the slaughter of 1.5 million chickens to stop H5N1 bird flu in its tracks, in spite of political opposition. She was vindicated. Her action was credited with bringing the epidemic under control.

In Helsinki, she laid it on the line. The speech on the dirty tricks of the food and drink industry, from the woman in charge of protecting and improving the world's health, is worth quoting at length.

'Efforts to prevent non-communicable diseases go against the business interests of powerful economic operators. In my view, this is one of the biggest challenges facing health promotion,' she said. '... It is not just Big Tobacco any more. Public health must also contend with Big Food, Big Soda and Big Alcohol. All of these industries fear regulation, and protect themselves by using the same tactics.

'Research has documented these tactics well. They include front groups, lobbies, promises of self-regulation, lawsuits, and industry-funded research that confuses the evidence and keeps the public in doubt.

'Tactics also include gifts, grants and contributions to worthy causes that cast these industries as respectable corporate citizens in the eyes of politicians and the public. They include arguments that place the responsibility for harm to health on individuals, and portray government actions as interference in personal liberties and free choice.

'This is formidable opposition. Market power readily translates into political power. Few governments prioritise health over big business. As we learned from experience with the tobacco industry, a powerful corporation can sell the public just about anything.

'Let me remind you. Not one single country has managed to turn around its obesity epidemic in all age groups. This is not a failure of individual willpower. This is a failure of political will to take on big business.

'I am deeply concerned by two recent trends. The first relates to trade agreements. Governments introducing measures to protect the health of their citizens are being taken to court, and challenged in litigation. This is dangerous.

'The second is efforts by industry to shape the public health policies and strategies that affect their products. When industry is involved in policy-making, rest assured that the most effective control measures will be downplayed or left out entirely. This, too, is well documented, and dangerous.

'In the view of WHO, the formulation of health policies must be protected from distortion by commercial or vested interests.'

There could not be a more powerful shot across the bows of the big corporations, nor a stronger warning to governments not to rely on industry's goodwill. WHO had fought a long battle with the tobacco industry and its allies before Chan took over. The lessons learned there have not been forgotten.

Sugar is the current whipping boy of the obesity pandemic, but there was an earlier villain – saturated fat. It was our love of butter and cream cakes, our passion for bacon and fat-marbled meat that was believed to be piling on the pounds as well as damaging our arteries.

When John Yudkin, the British scientist who published *Pure, White and Deadly* in 1972, started blaming sugar for harming health, he was out on a limb and earned himself the outright hostility of the sugar industry and its scientists. He found he was snubbed and passed over for research grants. In a second edition of his book, he wrote that while sugar was pure and white, the adjectives could hardly be applied to the behaviour of some of its supporters. Aubrey Sheiham, emeritus professor of dental health at UCL and a world authority on sugar and dental caries, knew Yudkin. He remembers a conference where the sugar-industry chair was so unpleasant when Yudkin stood up to speak, telling him in front of students that his work had been completely refuted, that he just sat down again without a word. 'He was so rude to Yudkin that my stomach turned. It was so obnoxious to insult this man in this audience,' said Sheiham.

Yudkin's hypotheses ran counter to those of Ancel Keys, an American biologist who first identified saturated fat as the enemy in the 1950s and whose work was thereafter hugely influential worldwide. Keys believed that heart disease was caused by a diet high in animal fat, while a Mediterranean-style diet in which olive oil was the main fat was protective. In his Seven Countries Study, investigating diet and heart deaths over 15 years in Finland, Greece, Italy, Japan, the Netherlands, United States, and Yugoslavia, he made a link between high cholesterol levels in the blood and heart disease. These findings had a major impact. The chase for the hare he set off led eventually to the development of statins, now very widely prescribed to people with high cholesterol levels, and multibillion dollar profits for drug companies. Some say the money and effort would have been better invested in promoting the Mediterranean diet that Keys himself backed.

Concern over dietary fat grew. In 1977, the US Senate committee on nutrition and human needs, better known as the McGovern committee, issued dietary guidelines for Americans. The Dietary Goals for the United States advocated less fat and cholesterol – as well as less sugar. Lobbying from farmers and the food industry succeeded in watering down the recommendations, but the 'fat is bad' message was the one that was remembered.

The food industry turned a setback into a sales opportunity. People were worried about fat – so give them low-fat products, which could be marketed as healthy. The shelves of supermarkets filled up with low-fat spreads and yoghurts and ready meals. But they were not necessarily less fattening. The calories from fat were replaced by calories from sugar and starches, which were needed to compensate for the loss of a creamy taste and texture.

'It didn't taste so good and you had to have some substance there,' said Harvard's Walter Willett. Refined starches were added to give bulk and sugar for taste. 'A lot of those products were really loaded up with sugar,' said Willett. 'That may have helped ratchet up our conditioning to a high level of sweetness.'

Based on this hypothesis that low-fat was good, the biggest, most expensive dietary study ever undertaken was launched. The Women's Health Initiative Dietary Modification Trial got underway in 1993, to test the effects of a low-fat diet, which many thought could end the obesity epidemic, as well as preventing some heart disease and cancers. There were high hopes. Nearly 50,000 women over the age of 50 were recruited, of whom 19,500 were put on a low-fat diet while the rest were encouraged to eat as they normally did.

But after eight years of low-fat food and counselling, the study, published in the *Journal of the American Medical Association*, found there were no benefits to a low-fat diet after all. It did not stop women putting on weight and nor did it prevent heart disease. There was a small reduction in breast cancers in the low-fat group, but not enough to be statistically significant.

There were the usual issues with the study, of course. The women on a low-fat diet may have not been entirely truthful about what they ate – or did not remember snacking between meals on cakes or burgers. As it was, they only reduced their fat intake from 38 per cent to 29 per cent instead of the 20 per cent which was the aim. That may go to show how difficult it is to eat a really low-fat diet, which means cutting down on high-protein food like meat and eggs as well as cheese and butter. Also, because they were between 50 and 79 years old, it may have been a bit late for the changed eating habits to have made a big impact on their health. But what is certain is that the experiment, costing hundreds of millions of dollars, was a failure.

Willett says that low-fat diets don't work for most people. They are unsatisfying. We are hungry soon after a low-fat meal. We go for high-carbohydrate foods to fill us up – too often the 'fast carbs' like sugar, white flour, white rice, potatoes and snacks. They give us a rapid spike in blood sugar and insulin levels, which is far from healthy.

It would be so good to point a finger at something we eat and say – that's it. That is what is making us fat. Then we could simply cut it out and get on with our more slender and healthy lives. I wondered what part our modern drinking habits are playing in the epidemic. Neither binge-drinking teenagers nor those in mid-life who like a gin before dinner and a bottle of wine or two with it think much about the calorie content. In fact, it's high. One large glass of wine is the calorie equivalent of four cookies, says Drinkaware, the alcohol industry-funded charity. A pint of lager is often the equivalent of a slice of pizza. How many of us factor that in? The NHS's National Obesity Observatory says alcohol accounts for 10 per cent of the calories of those who drink. It is energy dense – second only to fat and more than sugar.

But that's not all. Alcohol gives us the ultimate in empty calories. Because the body cannot store alcohol, the liver has to process it and get rid of it first. So the curry or the steak or the prawn risotto we have just eaten are put on hold and the calories they contain are more likely to be added to the fat stores than burned up. Glenis Willmott, leader of the Labour MEPs in the European Parliament, has been pushing to get calories added to wine, beer and spirit labels just as they are to food labels, against the opposition of the alcohol industry. But the way we drink and the reasons why we drink suggest that we will not be cutting down on beer and wine for the specific purpose of keeping our weight in check any time soon. We drink to have a good time and we drink to unwind from the pressure we are under in this fast-paced, ultra-convenient world, which offers us more food than we could possibly eat at affordably low prices.

So it's not simple. Sugar is a problem. Fat is a problem. Alcohol is a problem. They are all particularly problematic because they are energy dense, so contain a lot of calories – but it is too much of everything that is causing us the real trouble.

We are being misled by food companies. There are hidden sugars in our savoury meals and low-fat products are not always low in calories. It's there on the label, they argue, but you have to be obsessional about your weight to read all of the labels all of the time. Most of us are too busy to add up all the figures. And alcohol as yet doesn't have calorie labels anyway.

But there is a bigger problem still. Even if we make all the calculations, we sometimes don't and sometimes can't act on the information. It's not like making a rational decision to buy a car. We eat and drink to live and our emotions as well as physical pleasure are tangled up with food. And the food and drink companies know that very well.

3

ALL-DAY EATING

A metal hospital trolley, the standard variety with two shelves and a handle rail to push it along, is being loaded up, but not with drugs or dinner. No – this is the mid-morning snack trolley and it's being filled by two kind, elderly male volunteers at the WH Smith outlet in the reception area of the Royal Free Hospital in north London. They have put on some newspapers and a few useful toiletries. Now they are filling the rest of it with chocolate bars, crisps, biscuits, and cans and bottles of fizzy drinks. When they are done, they push the trolley, brimming with brightly coloured wrappers and calories, to the lift that will take them to the wards full of patients, some of whom will be suffering heart problems or diabetic complications as a direct result of a diet which includes too many of exactly these sort of snacks.

'That doesn't look very healthy,' I say as I walk with them along the corridor. Yes, replies one, some people have said that. But, he adds, 'If I was ill, I'd want a bit of a treat.'

And that is part of our problem. The snack trolley offers treats every day, just like all the sweet and snack and grocery stores at railway stations and bus stops on the way to work or to the park. Every day is treat day. Even when you are not ill, there is always going to be a reason why you deserve it. And the treats have got bigger. Chocolate once came in small portions. As a child, I used to be given a piece, not a whole bar. These days, we eat the slab in one. Who eats a single biscuit from a packet any more? Snack packs make it normal to eat several at a sitting. A snack is not a treat – it has become part of our daily routine. Anyone remember the advertising slogan, 'The sweet you can eat between meals without ruining your appetite'? The thought that chocolate bars might interfere with eating lunch or dinner enters nobody's mind any more. We have it all.

That mass consumption of snacks is why WH Smith in the Royal Free and everywhere else is no longer the book and newspaper store it used to be. It has a modest selection because people stuck in a hospital bed are likely to want to read. But the shelves fronting the reception area are full of sweets and other snacks and vibrant with purple and orange 'three for two' slogans on Cadbury products. This is where the money is now.

Cigarettes are banned in hospitals. Smoking is not allowed because it causes disease. But junk food, including the sort of snacks piled high on the trolley and demanding your attention in the reception area, is smiled on. Dr Aseem Malhotra, cardiology specialist registrar, is appalled and is campaigning for a ban. He won the support of the British Medical Association at its annual representative meeting in 2013. 'Hospitals have become a branding opportunity for junk food,' he told me. 'I'm not aware of any hospital that doesn't do it. It is perverse when we are telling people about healthy diets. Added sugar has no nutritional benefits.'

Yet it all started so well. The story of the origins of Britain's best-loved chocolate brand warms the heart. Around 120 miles north-west of the Royal Free, a model village was built at the end of the 19th century by a Quaker family in fields and by a wood said to be a relic of the Forest of Arden, to house the workers for their new factory four miles outside Birmingham. George Cadbury, chocolate maker, had high ideals for Bournville, which he hoped would 'alleviate the evils of modern more cramped living conditions'. The houses were designed in accordance with the ideas of the Arts and Crafts movement of William Morris and friends, with traditional-looking exteriors featuring mock-Tudor beams but plenty of space inside and large gardens. Cadbury wanted to improve not just the social conditions but also the mental and physical health of the people he employed. He was keen that Bournville's families should walk in the open air and play sport. Parks and recreational facilities were part of the original village design. Football and hockey pitches, an outdoor swimming pool filled from a natural mineral spring and a running track were built, together with a pavilion that functioned as both changing rooms and a social centre.

Bournville was about healthy living and chocolate was a part of the grand scheme of the Cadbury family for a better world – as well as a way to make money, of course. The original teetotal Quaker interest in cocoa was as a drink which might wean the populace off alcohol. It would be fair to assume that the Cadbury brothers, who launched their first chocolate bar in 1849 (two years after their fellow chocolate-making Quakers, the Fry family), never anticipated that their products could become a threat to health.

But Quaker philanthropists no longer run the chocolate industry. The company got bigger and merged with Schweppes and de-merged again; it bought soft drinks companies and gum companies and then eventually it was swallowed in 2010 by the vast US food company Kraft. The deal created much anger and anxiety in the UK, where Cadbury had been a beloved British institution, tied up with millions of British childhoods. Nobody ever really doubted that Willy Wonka's chocolate factory was in fact Cadbury's.

Kraft then spun off its 'snacking arm' into a new company it called Mondelēz. The name, which the company says was invented by an employee, is supposed to evoke both 'monde' – French for 'world' – and 'delight'. Somehow it doesn't have quite the Cadbury's magic.

Chocolate and sweets had already ceased to be a special treat by then. The TV advert that featured a balaclava-wearing James Bond-style hero fighting his way to his lady's bedroom to leave her a box of Milk Tray in the middle of the night would surely be risible now. Why didn't he pop into Smith's or Tesco or an all-night garage?

Mondelēz doesn't want it to be an effort to get hold of its chocolates, nor a rare event when we do. It wants its snacks to be part of our day, integral to our lives. It talks of 'three snacking needs', which it defines as 'treat, fuel and boost'. It offers us biscuits and cracker spreads for 'fuel' and its coffee brands for a 'boost'. Sweets fall into the treat category, defined in this way on the Mondelēz website: 'Chocolate, biscuits, gum and candy can lift our mood, giving us a moment of pleasure. We might feel we deserve a reward at the end of a difficult day and that a treat such as a piece of Cadbury or Milka chocolate, an Oreo biscuit or a stick of Trident Twist gum is just what we need to put a smile on our face.' The important words are the permissive ones – we 'deserve' it and we 'need' it. And modern consumption habits ensure the treat would be rather more than a single 'piece' of chocolate.

The snack companies use the most powerful weapon there is to market their products to us – not an appeal to our desire for health and wellbeing, but a hefty tug on our emotions. 'Every day we create delicious moments of joy,' says Mondelēz, which has nine billion-dollar brands (as well as very many smaller ones) marketed in 165 countries and revenue of $35 billion. 'We pour our hearts into creating snacks that treat, fuel and boost people worldwide.' The company is 'spicing different daily moments with delicious flavours and emotions'.

The interactive Cadbury Dairy Milk website – for the brand that decades ago used to be sold virtually as a health food, with 'a glass and a half of full-cream dairy milk' in every pound bar – is now called Joyville. It offers the Joyville story and the Joy-o-meter. It's not milk to make us grow strong that we are being offered today – it's happiness. The dice is loaded against us. How do we take responsibility for our weight and make rational decisions about what we eat when the food industry is playing our emotions?

Just how well the marketing of chocolate, sweets and cakes as treats works for the industry is clear from a Mintel marketing presentation to the Biscuit, Cake, Chocolate and Confectionery 2011 annual conference. Here Mintel's expert told the companies that they faced some challenges in hard economic times and that they were up against increasing pressure from health bodies. But on the positive side, said the slides:

'Half of UK consumers like to treat themselves to things they know are not good for them.

'A third of UK consumers buy chocolate on impulse.

'Despite concerns over fat and calorie content, adults like to reward themselves (and their kids) with sweets and chocolate.'

So that's all right then.

Mintel described this sector as 'a huge market', valued at about £9 billion (of which chocolate was £3.7 billion) and making up 7.5 per cent of total food expenditure. It forecast 30 per cent growth in the market from 2005 to 2015, when it would reach £10 billion.

Mondelēz is not the biggest snacking company in the world. That's PepsiCo – so much more than just a fizzy drink brand. Their snacking division in North America is called Frito-Lay, which manufactures, markets and sells corn chips, potato chips and other snack food. They own Walker's crisps, famously promoted in the UK by the popular and healthy-looking footballing commentator Gary Lineker.

Frito-Lay also sells with a pull on the emotions – this time not joy, but 'good fun!'

PepsiCo has been more responsive than most of the big food companies to the obesity crisis and criticism of junk food. Chief executive Indra Nooyi has attempted to shift the corporation in the direction of healthier products and has a research team working on low-calorie sweeteners. It has divided its products into three categories – good for you, better for you and fun for you (including Lay's potato chips, Walker's crisps, Doritos, Cheetos, Fritos and so on). There isn't one described as bad for you.

It's pretty hard to justify selling sugary sweets and drinks and salty, fatty crisps on health grounds, yet the snack food companies still try it. This is the argument they employ: eating small amounts all day long will cut your total calorie intake, they say, because you will not feel so hungry before your main meals. It's a clever sales pitch. This is how Mondelēz puts it: 'For many people, eating and drinking small amounts frequently throughout the day is part of a modern healthy lifestyle, a way they say helps keep both mind and body energised. We too believe that snacking can contribute to health and wellbeing, providing a flexible source of essential nutrients and energy. What's essential is to have a good overall balanced diet – and all foods can play a role in this.'

And this is Frito-Lay: 'Snacking is an important part of a balanced diet, whether you want to lose weight, sustain energy or simply live a better lifestyle. Snacking sensibly can curb your appetite between meals and keep your energy up during a busy workday.' It can be hard to know exactly how much you're eating, they add. That's why they sell their chips in single serving sizes, they say – and you can also buy '100 calories or less' packs.

In theory, it sounds plausible that a snack between meals might reduce our hunger for lunch or dinner when the time comes, with the result that we eat less, although most people – those outside the food industry and the governments that support it – would perhaps think a banana was a better idea than Oreos or Doritos or any other type of processed 'Os'. But does it really work that way?

Not according to nutritional expert Professor Barry Popkin. Snacks do not replace big meals – they add to them, he says. 'Snacking is a whole new behaviour,' he told me. 'Candy bars or soft drinks – that's about adding calories to your diet.

'Generally speaking, few countries in the world have any history of snacking before the second world war, except on a New Year's or some special holiday kind of occasion. A snack is a newly created behaviour. I think it's a combination of the industry, certainly, and higher income and the prevalence of food all around us. Whether you go to a grocery or a clothing store there is always some food and drink.

'Industry sees it as a growth sector, because they can get people to eat more times a day. That is part of the reason why Kraft spun off into Mondelēz, because snacking was the growth global business and Kraft US was kind of a traditional old cheese-and-other-kind-of-basic-food industry. And that's why Pepsi is one of the biggest snack companies in the world and Kellogg and all the big cereal companies see snacking as the growth sector.'

Cereal is no longer just for breakfast. Snack bars like Nutri-grain and grain-based desserts have hit the big time, he says. 'It is moving up in our countries – probably three-quarters of people don't cook or bake any more, they just buy these ready-to-eat desserts and snack on them as well as eat them at other times.'

The argument that snacks help you avoid over-eating at meal times does not wash, in his view. A study he published in 2010 in the journal *Health Affairs* showed that children in the USA are now eating almost contin-uously. On average, they were eating almost three snacks a day, as well as all their meals. 'Our children are moving toward constant eating,' wrote Popkin and his colleague Carmen Piernas, who looked at the changing eating habits of 31,000 children aged from two to 18 between 1977 and 2006. In 1977 a quarter did not eat between meals. That had completely changed by 2006, when almost all – 98 per cent – snacked. They ate more salty snacks like crisps and crackers and more candy and they drank more sweet-ened drinks. Over the 30 years, their calorie intake from snacks rose on average by 168 calories a day. Worryingly, the increase in snacking calories among the youngest children, aged two to six years old, was the highest – at 182 calories. And milk, fruit and vegetables had been replaced by sports drinks, fruit juice, cakes, sweets and biscuits.

'Kids still eat three meals a day, but they're also loading up on high-calorie junk food that contains little or no nutritional value during these snacks,' Popkin commented at the time.

The following year, 2011, he had a further paper published in the medical journal *PLOS Medicine*, which tried to pin down what it is about the way we adults eat that has led to the steady increase in our calorie intake – and the rise of obesity. Could it be that we are eating food that is just more fattening, or that we load our plates up in a way that we did not in the past or is it the number of times in the day that we eat? All three things had contributed to some extent, but the number of eating occasions – more and more snacks as well as meals – was the biggest issue of all, they found.

Data from the US Department of Agriculture confirms the snacking trend. In 2012, an analysis by the Agriculture Research Service showed that men and women were getting up to a third of their calorie intake from snacks with little or no nutritional value. Of the 5,000 men and women in the survey, which is published every two years, the men were consuming an average of 923 empty calories a day and the women 624. The ARS says that means men are consuming two to three times and women two to four times their recommended limits for fat and sugar per day. That's a lot of crisps, biscuits, sweets, cakes and fries in between proper meals.

We're talking effectively about all-day eating. There are no more social taboos about munching on the street, which my mother considered horrifying, or on public transport in front of dozens of strangers. Food smells assault us on trains and buses as fellow passengers tuck into chips or fried chicken without a second thought. Eating is now a function and an act of self-gratification that has nothing to do with anybody else.

We used to eat big meals, but we only ate three times a day, says Jane Ogden, professor of health psychology at Surrey University, who specialises in eating behaviour and obesity. 'My grandparents would have eaten a lot. My gran would have cooked my grandpa a big breakfast, he would have then come home for a proper lunch and then for a proper evening meal, whereas we have light breakfasts, a sandwich for lunch and then a big evening meal. But he would never have eaten in between those times – he wouldn't have dreamed of it and also he would have been on his feet. He would have walked to and from work and then whilst he was at work he would never, ever have sat down,' she told me.

Anna Soubry, the public health minister in the UK coalition government who was lambasted for saying obesity was an affliction largely of the poor, has also criticised the eating habits of working Britain. We have a 'weird' relationship with food, she said in January 2013, buying cookery books and watching TV chefs but not taking the time to prepare or eat good meals ourselves. And she was very damning about the typical office worker's lunch. 'It's disgusting eating over a keyboard,' she said. A lunch break ought to be an opportunity for people to 'chill out, get your head back together, and enjoy what you're eating', she told the *Daily Mail*.

Three months later, Soubry attacked Britain's snack culture in a debate in the House of Commons.

'Let us talk about something that did not exist when I was young – the concept of snacking,' she said. 'I was positively told not to eat between meals. If we now look in the real world at how young people live and at what they feel is acceptable, it includes going into the many coffee shops that exist. I have no problem with coffee shops, but young people go in and have a large coffee – not a small one … which has syrup in it. It might have marshmallows on top, and then perhaps another little dollop of cream, because it is just a snack, a treat or elevenses. "And by the way," they say, "I think I'll have one of those very nice muffins." They do not know how many calories that is. I absolutely agree that they do not understand that … That is why I absolutely congratulate all those places that have put up on their boards the number of calories in different foods.'

In a rare moment of accord across the party political divide, Soubry said that Labour's shadow public health minister, Diane Abbott, was right to suggest as she had in the debate that 'it is a surprise to people – even to supposedly intelligent, grown-up people such as ourselves – when they find out the calorific content of foods that we see and perceive as treats and snacks.' The two opposing politicians agreed that we really don't count snacking as part of our daily food intake.

But wary of suggesting there is anything intrinsically wrong with muffins and syrup in your coffee, Soubry then attempted to do a double-backflip and once more espouse the pro-food industry, government line. 'I want to make it clear that we should never demonise any food. There is nothing wrong with chips or burgers; what is important is that it is all good food in moderation,' she said. That throws the onus back on us. Resist temptation. Close your eyes to the emotional marketing ploys of the food industry. No help there from government.

The food industry continues to argue that snacking can reduce your appetite – and even help you lose weight. In 2013, the British Nutrition Foundation produced a review paper on snacking, written by members of its staff. It nodded to Popkin's work but suggested that what he had found in the US might somehow be different from the situation in the UK and Europe. It generally found the evidence for any link between snacking and obesity to be lacking. By the end of the paper, the foundation, which takes money from all the big food corporations, was positively endorsing snacking, saying that 'for some individuals, including young children, snacking may have a positive rather than negative impact on health and should not be discouraged on a population-wide basis'.[1]

The company that funded the paper, PepsiCo, must have been delighted.

Mondelēz has been conducting its own research into snacking. Jane Ogden accepted an invitation from Mondelēz in 2013 to take part in a big international consultancy exercise, which was billed as finding ways for snack-food companies to be more socially responsible in the face of the obesity epidemic.

'They interviewed me and that was fine and I basically told them that they should stop making snack foods, actually – if they wanted to behave morally, that was the way forward,' she told me. 'But if they still wanted to make a profit, given that they are a profit-making organisation, they should at least make healthy snack foods. I said if that involves bagging up apples, then fair enough. If you think you can con people to pay more for an apple because it's in a bag than an apple on its own, then that's your responsibility, but at least make it genuinely healthy.'

Afterwards it occurred to her that she could perhaps persuade Mondelēz to pay for one of her students to do a PhD in how to encourage people to eat healthier snacks. She proposed the idea and after some email exchanges, eventually had a telephone conversation with a senior manager at Mondelēz. She was disturbed by the way the discussion appeared to focus on increasing the sales of the products the company already had.

'I was saying to him, hold on a minute: are you making healthier snacks or are you marketing your unhealthy snacks as healthy? And he said, well, the latter actually. I wrote it down. Then he said evidence shows that high levels of snacking are related to lower levels of obesity, so the more we get people to snack, the less their BMIs will be. I said, well, that's just not true. I guess the grazing communities where you just don't have meals – maybe people in the Kalahari Desert or something who are constantly on the move – are thinner, but grazing plus meals is not a good recipe for anybody.

'It was kind of odd. I found it quite shocking. I said at the end, you know, I would never work with BAT [British American Tobacco] and I feel like now I'm speaking to the tobacco industry. I said I find that really uncomfortable.

'I've got the notes that I took: their biggest competitor is fruit, grazing is better than snacking and meals. Increased BMI is related to lower amounts of snacking; and people have the right to eat snacks in between meals because it makes them feel good and boosts their mood and we have no right to take that away from them.'

When I spoke to Mondelēz, it was clear how different their world view was from Ogden's. They start from a different premise altogether. No, they wouldn't consider developing a healthy snack, said their spokesman, because they do not recognise the term. 'The idea that there is a healthy food and an unhealthy food has long been dismissed by the industry and health professionals as meaningless,' he said. 'I don't understand the term healthy snack. We would say chocolate is not unhealthy. It is higher in fat and sugar than some things, but we are not advocating we eat choc-olate all the time.' Bananas are high in sugar but nobody is saying we should not eat bananas, he went on. And what about bread? 'It is all about a healthy diet and how you consume those products.'

The company is not arguing that we should give up our regular meals for non-stop snacking, he said. But if you are snacking, Mondelēz have different products available for different times of the day. They have breakfast bars, for instance, as well as biscuits for your morning coffee (hopefully Kenco, which they also make) and chocolate with your afternoon tea – if that's how you like your snacks. It's all up to you. As far as obesity is concerned, 'we're absolutely committed to playing our part', he said. They were not stepping away from the debate but working with the government. They were signed-up members of the Responsibility Deal. They have cut portion sizes to 250g, removed trans fatty acids and introduced re-sealable packs so people feel less need to eat a whole bar of chocolate at once.

But Mondelēz has not signed up to the traffic-light system. Presumably, I suggested, that is because they would get a big red light on the front of their packages? Not necessarily, he said. 'A bag of Liquorice Allsorts is low in fat and salt,' he said, which would give it green lights for those nutrients. But they are, of course, extremely high in sugar. That was his point – that it was unhelpful to the shopper to have a mixture of red and green lights on the packet.

Some of us are more susceptible to the blandishments of the food-industry marketeers than others but very few of us are rational beings with total control over what we eat. Our upbringing and our emotions play a huge part in the decision to choose the salmon bagel or the slice of coffee cake. Ogden, author of *The Psychology of Eating*, says our earliest food experiences programme our likes and dislikes.

'The basic psychological mechanisms are there from the moment we're born, which develop our sense of taste preference and the reasons why we eat, when we eat. The way I always teach it – if you ask lay people why they eat they say it's because they like it and because they're hungry. But actually taste preferences and hunger – neither of those are particularly strong drivers in terms of biological factors,' Ogden told me.

There are three simple processes in the development of our appetite, she said. One is exposure and familiarity. 'The more foods we are exposed to of a particular type, the more we like them, so children in England like chicken nuggets and pizza and children in Japan like fish and rice and children in China like noodles – we don't have different taste buds from those children. It is purely a cultural exposure process, which then breeds familiarity which then breeds preference.'

The second is modelling. 'We watch our parents and peers and TV and role models and we learn to like what they like. So the biggest predictor of what you will eat is what your parents eat. Then when you go into your teens your peers become a bit more of a stronger pressure.'

The third is association. If as children we are told we will have pudding if we eat our vegetables, we learn that vegetables are boring and only important to us as a way to access pudding. Later, when we have free choice, we eat pudding but skip the vegetables.

'It sets the whole reward process from a very early stage – and the same thing for exercise and all our behaviours,' Ogden said. 'I remember sitting next to this woman in Pizza Express and her little girl was sharing this huge, fantastic ice-cream thing and she said, "Oh you are lucky, look at this, this looks wonderful." They were having a really lovely mother and daughter moment, with a spoon each, and they were tucking in and the mother says, "Oh, this is much better than that pizza, isn't it?" and "Well done," and then she says, "If you eat all this you can go in the buggy – you don't have to walk."

'That child is learning so much in what looks like a nice, warm moment. She is actually learning that ice cream's exciting, pizza is boring and walking is boring.

'Where obesity fits in is that we've learned to like certain foods which mostly might not be good for us and we're modelling from people around us who might already be overweight and then on top of that the world bombards us with cheap, easily accessible food that we eat on the go. We eat in the car, we eat walking down the street, we eat at our desks, and because we don't mark that out as meal time, we don't register it in the same way. We know that if you're not concentrating on your food it doesn't make you as full and it doesn't make the hunger go away because you don't remember – you don't code it as being a meal.'

Hunger, it seems, is not just the uncomfortable physical prompting of the body that the stomach is empty and more fuel is required. It appears to be just as much to do with what is going on in your head. Dr Suzanne Higgs, reader in the psychobiology of appetite at Birmingham University, carried out a fascinating study with a group of amnesiac patients, who were unable to remember anything for very long at all, including what they had just eaten.

'We gave them a full lunch – sandwiches, cake,' she told me. 'They ate as much as they wanted. We took away the remnants of the meal that they'd just eaten. We waited just

10 or 15 minutes. We came back. We offered them the same meal again. We had control people [non-amnesiacs] who said, "Oh no, no, no thank you – I don't want any more to eat." The amnesiac patients ate the same amount again. They ended up eating about 2,000 calories in one sitting. You think the food's in their stomachs. They should be feeling full. But I think it actually demonstrates the power of these cognitive mechanisms.'

This is not just about forgetful individuals – it is an insight into the eating behaviour of all of us. If we remember what we've recently eaten, we don't feel so hungry. But in the modern world, when we are constantly rushing about or have our minds permanently locked into our smart-phones, we tend to forget.

'Food memories have an inhibitory effect on our appe-tite,' said Higgs. 'We can link this back then to the modern food environment, because there are lots of things nowa-days that really are set up to distract us from what we're eating, whether that's eating at your computer, eating in the street, on the go or even perhaps just a general fast-food culture which means that we don't sit down and linger over our meals or savour them.

'So really you can see how there are links into some cross-cultural differences – for instance, there is always the thing about the French paradox, where the French seem to manage to get away with eating high-fat foods and they didn't used to have problems with obesity, although that is changing a little bit. But certainly there is the idea that you could just eat a little bit of something that's very tasty and perhaps the way in which you ate was important, not just what you eat.'

Higgs is now working on ways to prompt people about the food they have recently eaten, but may have forgotten about – such as a phone app, which you can use to take a photo of your lunch, which will then pop up as a reminder later on. Memory is important, but so is attention to what you are eating, she says. We need to enjoy our food, choose it carefully and take time over eating it. Perhaps it is time to think about scrapping TV dinners and bringing back the old-fashioned family meal.

'I'm not one to advocate going back to the good old days or old traditional values but actually I do think that is a conclusion from this work: that eating, sitting down, making time for that – and eating in company, that's great as well – I do think that there are advantages to that sort of eating pattern, that's for sure,' she said.

And snacking starts to look less and less smart. 'You might be doing that when you are doing something else – grabbing something, heading back to your desk with a doughnut. You talk to people about it as well and they say, "Well, yeah actually, I've done that before, where you've had a packet of sandwiches at the desk for lunch and you think you've only eaten half of them and actually you've eaten the whole thing without even realising it because you've been so distracted."'

How often do we ever really pay attention to what we are eating? Deborah Cohen of the Rand Corporation in California says that we do not naturally think too much about it. Eating is an 'automatic behaviour' – it is something people often do without over-exerting their consciousness. 'People are generally not aware of how much they are eating,' she says in her 2008 paper in the journal *Preventing Chronic Disease*. 'Once people initiate eating, they usually continue until the food is gone or until some other external occurrence changes the situation. In one study, people were less likely to stop eating because they were full than because no food or drink remained, they had no time to eat more, or they had finished watching television ... Effort is not required to continue eating when food is present; effort is required to refrain from eating when food is present.'

That doesn't mean we can't bring our behaviour under control, she writes. We are all capable of saying no to chocolates or dessert. 'All automatic behaviours can be controlled temporarily. Human beings can consciously prevent themselves from smiling when amused, frowning when annoyed, or tensing their muscles when threatened. It just takes effort. But the amount of effort required to refrain from eating when food is present is substantial, and it is nearly impossible to sustain over the long term.'

Keeping your weight down is just not that easy in an environment where there is too much easily available food and too many messages directed at us to try to persuade us to buy it and eat it, she says. In her book, *A Big Fat Crisis*, she further explores this idea that people are not in control of what they eat all the time and takes it to its logical conclusion. 'It is the environment we should be working on instead of trying to tell people to change their behaviours, because people's behaviours are only because of the way the environment is designed,' she told me.

'It is impossible to think self-control is really the problem. If you look around, you see all kinds of people having a problem with weight and obesity – doctors, nurses, PhDs in nutrition. It is not to do with what you know. I don't think it's self-control because it takes a lot of self-control to get a PhD.'

Food-industry marketing is aimed at undermining this precarious self-control. In an article in 2012 for the *New England Journal of Medicine* she cited the positioning of 'candy at the cash register', strategically placed there to encourage impulse buying.

'Impulse marketing works through the placement and display of products in retail outlets. In fact, the arrangement of products in stores is the most important malleable determinant of sales. For example, goods placed in prominent end-of-aisle locations account for about 30 per cent of all supermarket sales,' she wrote. 'Indeed, vendors pay a slotting fee to retail markets to guarantee that their products will be placed in these locations.'

Placing products prominently where shoppers cannot miss them may increase sales up to five times. Food marketing people test out the best places in or at the end of the aisles to put their sweets or biscuits using sophisticated machines that register exactly what draws the eye. The longer your glance holds it, the more likely you are to add it to your trolley. Big Brother is watching what you are watching.

Cohen thinks we are being menaced and frankly need protection. 'In general, buildings, cars, toys, and other products are designed to account for limits of human capacity. Although people could certainly stay away from the edges of balconies and not lean out of windows, mandatory railings and window guards protect them from falling in cases in which they may otherwise wander too close. With strong empirical research, it should be possible to identify which marketing strategies place people at risk or undermine their health, as well as to quantify the magnitude of risk. This kind of knowledge should be applied in informing regulations that could govern the design and placement of foods in retail outlets to protect consumers.'

Not the sort of academic to define the problem and then depart for an ivory tower, she is looking for funding to create a new type of supermarket, which would put healthy food in the prime locations and help people decide what to cook and guide them on what to buy. 'There'd be no candy at the cash register or chips in the aisle,' she told me, 'but also a lot of demonstrations of what the meals should look like. Supermarkets have got things all over the place. It is not easy for someone to figure out what their meal should look like. These huge supermarkets with 40,000 to 50,000 different items are totally unnecessary. We need fewer options than are available. They overwhelm people.'

It really is an unfair world. Many people who are overweight are well aware of this, as they watch their skinny friend demolish burgers and chips and snack on doughnuts. Some of us only have to look at a piece of cheesecake to gain weight. Others are lean for life.

So far only one actual 'fat gene' has been found, called FTO, but science is catching up with what appears to most people to be the blindingly obvious. Some people are programmed to be fat and others to be thin. It does not seem to be anything to do with the speed or efficiency with which different people's bodies process food. It may instead have a lot to do with the brain.

'I myself am convinced that the key psychological traits that are relevant to people becoming obese in the first place are to do with the way their appetite is structured and that is largely genetic,' said Professor Jane Wardle, a health psychologist at University College London.

There are people who are primed to become fat and people destined to stay thin, she thinks. That does not let the junk-food outlets and supermarkets off the hook. The fat-prone are their best customers – some people might call them their victims. People who put on weight are more responsive to food marketing – to the pictures and the aromas and the slogans inviting us to stop and buy and eat. They are also less likely to know that feeling towards the end of a big meal when you cannot eat another bite. The satiety mechanism doesn't function as fast or as fully or at all. So unlike their slimmer friends, they don't stop when the fuel tank is full.

'It would always have been valuable in populations to have people who can eat more,' says Wardle. While the skinny hunters were out running after animals, the plumper members of the tribe could gather food. And in lean times, when the food runs out, the fatter last longer.

Few of us were fat 50 years ago. Wardle muses on the difficulty of getting enough calories down you to last through the afternoon when you were subjected to cabbage for lunch at school. I couldn't agree more – I have a very clear memory of being made to sit in front of the semolina I was refusing to eat through most of the afternoon's first lesson. 'Food is ever nicer, nearer and cheaper,' she says. 'If you have got those genetic propensities, it is ever more likely you will express them.'

So much nicer, but the trouble is, there is just too much of it. We live in a time of feast. The food industry has for years produced more than we need and now they have to persuade us to keep on buying it, according to Professor Philip James of the International Association for the Study of Obesity, one of the world's leading experts. They push, promote and dangle food in front of us in a way they never used to when there was just enough to go round – and he blames them for deliberately disrupting the old, social, three-meals-a-day eating habits.

'Now why did the epidemic take off in 1980? I believe it took off because of the brilliant new understanding of how to go about marketing. By marketing, I mean the selling of surplus food.

'We produce 50 per cent more food than we need, so by definition all the companies were having to find ways to sell their produce. It's not very complicated. You could say the increase in snacks, the increase in soft drinks, these are all methods by which you disrupt the normal eating of food. It is ideal to get people away from eating meals sitting around the table because there, you have select episodes and you have to prepare the food and it's all semi-controlled, whereas when you're in a free-for-all, then any stimulus will lead to subconscious instinct [and] emotional repetitive responses.'

The more food that is available to us, the more we eat. Look at the rise and rise of the buffet meal, he says. It happened because hotels realised buffets were a huge opportunity to cut their costs, but for us, they mean bigger plates of food.

'If you have a buffet, you eat 20 per cent more than you would eat if you were served your meal,' he said. 'And think of how many waiters you need [for customers served at tables] compared with four people keeping that buffet going. That's an enormous saving that totally outweighs the cost of that 20 per cent more food.'

The temptation to eat more than normal is almost irresistible. If we eat too much of the same thing, the taste begins to pall. We are bored with it. We have what Barbara Rolls described as 'sensory-specific satiety'. But the variety offered at a buffet overcomes that problem. We can eat and eat because each new helping tastes different and exciting.

But our social conditioning also plays a part. A buffet is a social meal, where we are queuing for food and selecting our helpings alongside other people. Most of us do not want to appear greedy. 'If you put on the end of the buffet small plates and large plates and the person before you picks up the small plate, you are much more likely to follow with a small plate. If they then put two heaps of rice on it, you are much more likely to go for two rather than four,' said James. Unfortunately, of course, the converse is also true.

We go with the pack. So it is more than easy for the food industry to get us to eat more or more often. All they have to do is normalise frequent snacks or big portions. Supersize me? Certainly. A tub of popcorn at the cinema that is almost bigger than your child? Of course – everybody else has one. When it comes to food, we are likely to do what the rest of the herd does.

Undoubtedly we could do with better information about what is in our food. It has been a struggle to get labelling that clearly gives us an idea of how much fat, salt and sugar a ready meal or packet of biscuits contains, but the coalition government eventually embraced the red, green and amber colour-coding notion that Labour dodged. Under the Responsibility Deal, Starbucks has agreed to put calories on the menu in the UK, as have over a third of restaurants and takeaways.

Whether anybody takes much notice is another matter. A study before and after New York introduced menu calorie labelling in 2008 found that only one in six customers used the information to make a healthier choice. Looking for calories on the menu boards at a British motorway service station, at first I thought Starbucks did not display them, but eventually noticed small, faded figures, almost too small to read, beside the price. KFC's board was more legible and McDonald's the best, with calorie counts in boxes beside each item – but you would have to be actively looking for them. In the distraction of the array of meals and deals and prices, when you are hungry and possibly in a hurry, the calories are the last thing you notice. And it is only the big chains that have agreed to display calories. The other one-off cafes selling fast food at the service station did not.

Labelling is a really good thing, but it is no simple solution. It works for those people who are overweight and have determined that they will lose some pounds. Most of us don't think to look or we are in too much of a hurry. We grab food and go and then forget what we've eaten, feel hungry and grab some more. Obesity is one of the penalties for the crazy way we live today, in a hurry, racing from one task to the next. And it's about the environment around us that has developed to allow us to step up the pace in this way. That's the justification for fast food – to help us live life in the fast lane – and snacks – to keep up our energy (and give us fun and joy, of course).

We don't have time for anything, which is why we graze on the go rather than sit down to proper meals. It's also why we jump in the car rather than walk, and drive it to the supermarket where we can load up quickly before racing home to – well, probably watch the TV out of exhaustion at the speed of our lives.

So we will be making snap decisions at Tesco or Asda, where we are faced with mountains of choice and a wall of brightly coloured wrappers and enticing packaging grabbing our attention and urging us to reach for the easiest options – the sweets, chocolate, crisps and cereal bars that now make up such a large proportion of our shopping baskets.

Given all the extra calories we are consuming via snacks, we need to be more active. There is no doubt that our increasingly sedentary lifestyle, locked to a computer screen during the day and a TV screen in the evening, is part of the reason why so many of us have put on so much weight. People who might have had manual jobs in the past involving heavy physical work would have eaten large, calorific meals and had not an ounce of excess fat on them.

The Foresight report in 2007 put figures on it. Over the previous 30 years, it said, physical activity had 'declined significantly'. The average distance walked by people in England to get from one place to another – as opposed to strolling for the fun of it – dropped from 255 miles a year in 1975 to 192 miles in 2003. Cycling was similarly hit, with the annual average mileage down from 51 miles to 34 miles in the same time period. Meanwhile car use rose by 10 per cent. A fifth of all journeys of less than one mile were made in the car.

Most people used to get their physical exercise either through the work they were doing, whether washing clothes by hand or digging in the fields, or by walking or cycling miles to their job or to the shops (and carrying heavy bags of groceries home). But nobody wants to turn the clock back. We like our cars and our modern, technology-enhanced lifestyle. Those who say physical exercise is the answer often go against the grain of modern life. Even getting off the bus at an earlier stop, so that we walk a mile on the journey to work, is an unwelcome suggestion when time is tight and people are commuting for longer distances than ever before.

More sport and physical leisure activities would obviously be good for us, but research tends to show that it is the more affluent who engage in it. 'Deprivation and poverty were found to be associated with low levels of leisure-related physical activity in a number of studies,' said Foresight.

It can help, though, to live in a town that has been planned and designed with walking and cycling in mind – so that it becomes a quicker and easier option to go down the road to the local shops on foot and there are green spaces, cycle lanes, activities and sports facilities near people's homes and cars are made less welcome. In fact, the Cadbury brothers probably had it about right when they built Bournville. Unfortunately, today's towns and cities very rarely look like Bournville. They look a lot more like Tamworth and Gateshead, two of the first boroughs in the UK where more than 30 per cent of the population are officially obese.

4

THE FATTEST TOWNS IN BRITAIN

On a bench in Market Street in Tamworth, Staffordshire, facing the Fat Sandwich shop on a bitingly cold winter day, sit a man and a woman eating pasties out of paper bags. Both are very large – there is no need for a set of bathroom scales to figure out that they are several times the healthy weight for their height. When they finish, the man heaves himself up with difficulty to throw the wrappings into a nearby bin. The woman leans heavily forward onto the crutches she needs for support, preparing to go. Neither smiles nor looks in the least bit happy. Neither speaks. It did not appear to be a very pleasurable meal.

But at least lunch didn't cost them much. Fast food and takeaways are not pricey in Tamworth. The Fat Sandwich sells bacon baguettes for £1.99 and sausage baguettes even more cheaply, for 99p. It undercuts the large van, engine humming, planted on the pedestrianised street opposite, which sells burgers for £2. Up the road is Greggs, the cake and pastries shop that had a moment of fame in 2012 when Chancellor George Osborne slapped tax on microwave-heated pasties and then backtracked in the hullaballoo that followed. He was forced to admit that he could not remember when he last bought a pasty in Greggs and tried to duck charges that he was too posh to set foot inside, while prime minister David Cameron claimed to have eaten one at a railway station. In Tamworth, the shop is doing a roaring trade.

Fast food is not only cheap here but plentiful. McDonald's may have moved out of the centre into the large residential district of Wilnecote, a couple of miles to the south, but it now has a drive-through for ultimate convenience. No need to walk. Could all of this have anything to do with the average girth of the population? The couple on the bench in the town centre are far from untypical. Tamworth, once famous as the home of the Reliant Robin, the three-wheeler car invented in Tom Williams' back garden here in 1935, is now notorious as the fattest town in England.

According to the National Obesity Observatory, the government's official source of data, which analysed the statistics in the Health Survey for England, more than 30 per cent of the adult population of Tamworth was obese in 2011. The Staffordshire market town tied for first place in the fat league table with Gateshead on 30.7 per cent. Two more boroughs, Swale and Medway in Kent, also topped 30 per cent obesity, at 30.2 per cent and 30 per cent respectively.[1]

Inhabitants of the four districts may have felt unfairly stigmatised, but the 30 per cent figure was highly significant. The Foresight report of 2007, commissioned by government to map the scale of the problem facing Britain and suggest the way forward, warned that 60 per cent of UK men and 50 per cent of women would be not just over-weight but actually obese by 2050 if nothing was done. Various initiatives have followed, but while the steady rise in adult obesity has slowed, the trend is ever upwards.

The four boroughs named by the NOO were the first in the country to break the 30 per cent ceiling. To walk through Tamworth is to step into the Fat Britain of the future. Where this town has gone, the rest of the country is also going. Tamworth has just been forced to wrestle with the issues of obesity ahead of many other local authorities in the UK.

All around you in the dignified red-walled town centre are reminders of the glorious and much thinner past. Tamworth is a small and very English market town, over-looked by a modest Norman castle. In the middle of Market Street is its elegant old town hall, built on sturdy Tuscan-style stone pillars, which used to enclose the butter market and where the fire engine was later parked. It was erected in 1701 by Thomas Guy, book publisher, stock speculator and at one point MP for Tamworth, who went on to found Guy's Hospital in London.

In front of the town hall is the large (but well-proportioned) statue of one of England's great Victorians, Sir Robert Peel, famous to the nation as the creator of the 'bobbies' or 'peelers', precursors of the modern police force, and locally as the original breeder of the Tamworth pig. Peel, who was initially elected as MP in the 'rotten borough' of Cashel, Tipperary, took over the Tamworth seat at his father's death in 1830, four years before his first period as prime minister. He relinquished it only at his death in 1850 following a fall from a horse – it was a rather more active era than ours.

If Peel were looking around his constituency today, he might well be taken aback. There are no more skinny, underfed Victorian urchins ready to scamper up narrow chimneys, that is for sure. Tamworth is visibly, undeniably fat. In the small Ankerside shopping centre which opens off Market Street, many people in late middle age walk slowly and with apparent difficulty, shifting their weight painfully from one leg to the other. A good many have sticks. Others can no longer walk and get about on motorised scooters, propelling their bulk gently and without any physical exertion past Peacocks, the Body Shop, mobile phone outlets and other chain stores that have ousted the butcher, greengrocer and baker that Peel's freezer-deprived constituents would have walked to each day.

Peel would notice the difference, but it is strange how quickly the brain adjusts to the surroundings and the eye ceases to see it. Local GP John James remarks on how perceptions have changed. Nobody appears obese in films from the 1950s and children in photographs of the era seem to us to be stick-thin, he says. Yet they are of normal weight. We have just got used to seeing fatter people.

'I have been a GP for 30 years,' said Dr James, based in next-door Lichfield and chair of the clinical commissioning group for the whole area. 'When I was a student, we were talking about the average British male being a man of 70 kilos [11 stone].

'We don't need the statistics. We have all seen it happen. But we normalise visually. We look around the room at other people and say, "I'm fairly tall or I'm not very tall."' So when most people are fat, fat appears the norm.

Tamworth's councillors, officials and dignitaries were not best pleased with its nomination as the fattest town in the country and argue with some justification that the tag is unfair. The data on which it was based was the latest available, but it was from 2006 to 2008 and the obesity percentages are estimates. Tamworth's score was not, of course, greatly different from that of neighbouring towns and that is clear from the regional data published by the National Obesity Observatory. The fattest region overall was the north-east, which includes Gateshead, where 27.8 per cent of people were obese, and then the West Midlands, which includes Tamworth, on 26.4 per cent. London had the least obesity, at 20.7 per cent, although that ranged from skinny and well-to-do Kensington and Chelsea on 13.9 per cent to Barking and Dagenham on 28.7 per cent.

But although they cry foul and contest the accuracy of the figures, as well as pointing to everything they are doing now to slim down the population, Tamworth's leaders do not dispute that they have a problem. 'We can run around saying the figures are out of date, but the bottom line is there is still an obesity issue,' said Councillor Jeremy Oates, who sits in the council's cabinet and has health as part of his remit.

So why is Tamworth one of the fattest places in England? If there were simple answers, says district public health lead

Jonathan Topham, they could probably sort it out. 'It is so multi-faceted, we can't be sure,' he said.

Tamworth had a population of only 7,000 in 1931. Its big growth spurt came from the 1960s on, when the boundaries were expanded and people working in Birmingham, 14 miles away, began to move out of the city in search of cheaper homes and views of green fields. In 2010, there were 76,000 people living in the town, with a high population density. Tamworth is now classified as 100 per cent urban.

The largest proportion of the population in 2010 were 55- to 64-year-olds. This is a post-war baby boom generation and they have just hit the age at which health problems really kick in. A survey of a sample of GP practices showed that one in four people had some sort of long-term medical condition and a third of those were obese. The biggest cause of death is already heart disease.

Tamworth is not a rich town. Manufacturing has declined across the Midlands and most jobs are now in service industries. Wages are not high. But less than 3 per cent of the working population are unemployed. Some parts of the town are worse off than others, but it is hard to argue that poverty in Tamworth is the only reason for the size of so many of its people.

Staffordshire county council and the local NHS use the Mosaic system to categorise the local population – a geo-demographic system developed in the 1980s, but refined over the years, which slots us all into social groups with titles that might have some of us up in arms if we only knew how we had been categorised. According to the Tamworth health profile, the largest proportion of residents (18 per cent) fall into the 'Suburban Mindsets' group, described as 'manual and white collar, married, middle age, children, leafy suburbs, comfortable affordable housing, home improvement, family life, industrious, [and shopping for] mainstream brands'. Just behind that are 'Industrial Heritage' who are 'traditional, married, below average incomes, approaching retirement, outgrown homes, personal responsibility, manufacturing industries, careful with money, reliant on cars, manual skills'. Nine per cent are 'Claimant Cultures', defined as 'disadvantaged, low incomes, unemployment, long-term illness, low-rise council housing, one-parent families, high TV watching, dependent on state'.

Tamworth, in common with anywhere else, has its prosperous and poorer parts.[2] Interestingly, in spite of the general assumption that it is poor people who are obese, the Tamworth health profile shows that there is little difference between the prevalence of obesity across differing-income areas of Tamworth.

It is so easy to assume that excess weight is a problem of poor people. That's not true in Tamworth or anywhere else. There are overweight people in every strata of society, even if the numbers are higher amongst those who have less money. In fact, an interesting study carried out in Leeds found that it was not how much money you had, but where you lived that made the difference.

Dr Claire Griffiths and colleagues from Leeds Metropolitan University looked at children's obesity by postcode. Their results – published in February 2013 – revealed that the biggest proportion of fat children lived in areas of 'middle affluence' – in other words, neither the richest nor the poorest areas. They don't know for sure what to make of their findings, but whether it is public transport or bike lanes, fresh food shops or cheap takeaways, something about the particular streets a child lived in made him or her more likely to put on weight or stay thin.

Rob Barnes, director of housing and health in Tamworth, says he thinks part of it is about what people know, what they have learned and what they choose to eat or do with their lives as a result. 'There is a link between unhealthy lifestyles and educational attainment and aspiration,' he said.

Tamworth does not score well on education. It had the lowest proportion of young people in Staffordshire attaining five or more A*–C GCSE grades (including English and Maths) in 2011 – 49 per cent compared with nearly 56 per cent across the county. 'Areas of low educational attainment and skills are often associated with high levels of worklessness, deprivation and poor health,' states Staffordshire's 2012 joint needs assessment strategy document.

The town also has high rates of teenage pregnancy – in fact the sixth highest conception rate among 15- to 17-year-old girls in the country in 2010 and still rising. Breastfeeding rates are low and smoking rates, at 25 per cent of the population, are the highest in the county. All of those things also tend to increase amongst those who have failed – or been failed – at school.

Tamworth, like everywhere else, has a car culture, even if it no longer features Reliant Robins, which ceased production in 2001. There are bike lanes and paths where people can go jogging, but generally people do not walk to the butcher, baker and greengrocer of Peel's era on a daily basis any more – who does? The weekly shop is done at a supermarket, by car. The Active People Survey of 2009/10 asked residents about 250 different types of sports and leisure pursuits, including dancing and gardening, and yet only 9 per cent of men and women in Tamworth could say they met the recommended levels of physical activity. That was similar to the national average, but almost three in five (57 per cent) men and women were completely inactive – not even taking a weekly walk or weeding the garden. That is significantly higher than the national average. They have low scores on healthy eating as well, measured by fruit and vegetable intake. Only 22 per cent of people in the town eat five pieces of fruit or portions of vegetables a day, which is worse than the average (29 per cent) for England.

'We do have issues around lifestyle and behaviours,' said Topham. 'We have lower levels of physical activity than you would expect. It looks like the levels of healthy eating are not as good as they should be. They are probably the lowest in the county. There is probably a correlation with obesity.'

So could it be that the fault lies with the pasties, buns and burgers bought and eaten in Tamworth's streets instead of oranges and bananas – or indeed the Japanese sushi or other healthy (and expensive) foreign delicacies that you might see highly educated, aspirational folk choosing in England's most affluent town centres?

The National Obesity Observatory carried out a study to see whether the most deprived local authorities had the greatest density of fast-food outlets. Tamworth has 64 per 100,000, which is fairly modest and well short of Gateshead's score of 97. But, on the other hand, more affluent and educated South Cambridgeshire has only 15 per 100,000 and West Devon has 28. And the fast-food outlets counted were limited to takeaway and delivery outlets like burger bars and fish and chip shops. Cake and pasty shops were not included.

Certainly local people blame burger bars. When the council convened a Citizens' Panel, said Topham, 'we asked whether people thought obesity was an issue and if so, why? Fast food and the proliferation of places like McDonald's and KFC and fish and chip shops are the first things people say.' They also tended to believe that people on lower incomes were more likely to be obese and either didn't know about nutrition or have any cooking skills or else did not have the money to eat well. 'There is a perception that money is a barrier towards being physically active or healthy eating,' he said.

It is true that lack of money means you can't afford a Saturday afternoon at the SnowDome – more evidence of Tamworth ingenuity, it is the first indoor ski slope in Britain with real, machine-made, snow. Walking and playing football in the park are free, but motivation is in short supply on cold and rainy days when the sofa and the TV look more inviting.

But on a wander round Tamworth, it was pretty clear that fat was not limited to people with little money. With over 30 per cent obesity, it cannot be so.

The wonderfully named Silk Kite pub, recalling a dangerous experiment Benjamin Franklin carried out in 1752 involving flying a kite attached to a metal key in an electrical storm, offers plentiful but not cheap food in an attractive Art Deco building from the 1930s. The menu outside lists the calories of every meal: a cheese and ham toastie is 448 calories, a club sandwich 750 calories and a British Beef and ale pie weighs in at a substantial 1222 calories – half the daily recommended intake for a man (2605) and more than half that of a woman (2079). Whether the clientele, with sufficient money to eat there, knew or cared is questionable. Unless the windows were made of that fairground magnifying mirror glass, all appeared to be at least twice the size they would want to be if they had real concern for their health.

What could or should Tamworth's leaders do about the swelling girth of its population? GP John James points out that the first problem is to dare to raise it with anybody who is overweight. He tells the tale of a patient who came to his practice and saw one of his colleagues. 'He said to me, "I don't like your mate. He told me I was obese." I said, "Well, you are a big lad." He said, "Yes, I'm fat, but I'm not obese,"' said James. The F-word was acceptable to him, but the O-word was not. Fat can be puppy-fat. Fat can be a joke. Obese sounds to many people like a term of abuse.

'We have got to find a language,' said James, who draws parallels with smoking. In the 60s, it was normal to smoke, he says. You felt embarrassed to ask somebody not to light up in your house. That has utterly gone.

James admits he is probably in a minority of GPs in speaking to his patients about their weight when they come in for other reasons, such as problems with their knees or their feet. If he does raise it, he says, they are usually receptive. 'The vast majority of my grossly obese patients – even the obese ones – want to do something about it. I have never sat down and really tried to tease out what is stopping them doing it. I think it's societal pressure.'

He says he thinks GPs could maybe help people to make healthy choices about their food – advise them not to drink copious amounts of cola or eat pasties and chips all the time – in the same way that they were able to tell people it was a good idea, regardless of the behaviour of their friends and relatives, to give up the fags.

'Sometimes it is about enabling people – saying it is acceptable to make healthy choices. We have been reticent, but as GPs we are getting more comfortable at saying to people your weight is going to become an increasing problem for your health,' he says.

Not everybody has a GP who is prepared to use even the F-word with them. Michelle Wright was 47 years old, 5 feet 6 inches tall and weighed over 100kg (16 stone) when she went to see her GP with pains in her joints and her feet. 'My doctor didn't even say to me I was overweight,' she said. 'He just started me on steroid injections. He didn't advise me to lose weight or anything.'

She knew herself that she was too heavy. 'At Christmas last year I was in size 22s. My Christmas present under the tree was the biggest parcel there and when I opened it, it was a coat,' she said. It was huge. Something had to change, she decided.

Wright started trying to cut the calories in the food she ate on her own, but then saw adverts for Weight Watchers in the New Year and joined up. 'When I lost about 20kg (3 stone), the pain stopped in my feet,' she said.

She thinks the epidemic of overweight – which she believes is no different in Tamworth from anywhere else – is down to the pressures on the consumer today. 'I really do,' she said. 'You only have to sit down and watch TV. There are the special offers, buy one get one free, boxes of Maltesers in the supermarket for £1. But also people are making the wrong choices. It is down to willpower as well. You choose what you put in your mouth.'

She used to be, she says, a pie and chips person. Her children are now 18 and 20, so there is no more routine cooking and eating of an evening meal all together. Most people are too busy, she adds, working 45 hours a week. Convenience foods save time.

But she mentioned something else, which kept appearing in the stories I heard from people who are or have been overweight. It is unhappiness, either as the cause or as an effect of becoming fat. Wright says that she was aware of it when she was putting on weight. 'I think I was unhappy with myself. As you put weight on, you start to think, "This is the way I'm going to be." It is about self-esteem. You get to a certain point and you think, "This is me, now." This time last year I was a very, very sad person with no self-esteem. But you can do something about it.'

Wright has lost more than 30kg (5 stone) through eating better food, including far more fruit and vegetables, and exercising by walking her dog. She is now a dress size 12, but keeps the coat to remind her of the way she was, as well as a pair of trousers because she can now get both legs into one. She has learned to 'make sure you are thinking why you want to eat – because you are hungry or thirsty – or bored or because you saw a chocolate bar advert? It is a big, big mind game.'

Anne Devenney's weight gain was most definitely the result of emotional distress. Her fourth child, Cameron, was diagnosed with a very rare blood disorder when he was 15 months old, after four months of tests. He needed a bone-marrow transplant. All three of his siblings were a match and his five-year-old brother donated, but Cameron suffered complications after the operation and eventually died.

'He was in Birmingham Children's Hospital for virtually six months,' she said. 'It became ready meals and hospital meals and never leaving the room because he was in isolation. We [the parents] called it the mum's shuffle – wandering down the corridor in your slippers.'

Devenney's weight went up to 103kg (16 stone 4 lb) and she had to wear size 20 clothes. She used to order two big breakfasts at the McDonald's drive-through and eat both. 'I can't face even one now. You get a little bit embarrassed because you feel disgusted that you did that.

'People don't necessarily understand how difficult it can be. Even now I can still have bad days and revert to the old eating pattern. I'm still in danger of reaching for that chocolate. I don't think that will ever leave me.'

There came a point when she knew she had to do something. At the children's hospital, she used to have to leave her car on the sixth floor of a multi-storey car park. 'There were six flights of steps. I struggled to get up there. I used to have to do a couple and stop and I was nearly in tears because I felt so ashamed at how I'd got.'

In the end, she knew she had to act for the sake of her other children. 'It was a good few weeks after we'd lost him. I was eating a lot and down with everything. Then it was a sudden realisation that I didn't want a tragedy for the others. If I carried on, they were going to have another tragedy. I looked at myself and felt dreadful.'

A friend took her walking to get her out of the house. One night she saw a group of women from an athletics club running and decided that was what she wanted to do. With the support she got from her Slimming World group, she ate better food, brought her weight down to 67kg (10 stone 8 lb) and is now a size 10 – and a keen runner.

What made it all possible for her was support, she says. 'It is really hard for people unless they have that. I suppose some can do it on their own, but long term it has to be about lifestyle change. It is not down to what people think of as greed, even if it's a case of over-eating. There's always something else behind it.'

When it comes to weight, your friends really matter. They can help you lose weight or they can help you put it on. We are sociable creatures. We tend to take on the habits, the likes and dislikes and norms of the people around us. Surveys have shown that people who are overweight often have friends who are overweight. The Framingham Heart Study in 2007 showed that your chances of becoming obese rose by 57 per cent if a friend became obese. That went up to 71 per cent if the friend was of the same sex. Friends had far more influence than husbands and wives – but after all, not many of us consider our spouse a role model.

Devenney thinks genetics play a part too. 'I have two children who will stop when they are full but one who will eat like me,' she said. Did she not stop eating when she was full? She laughed. 'The trick was to eat it fast. I did read somewhere that people who are overweight don't necessarily enjoy food. When I thought about it, I used to eat so fast I probably didn't even taste the food. It was the sheer sensation rather than savouring it.'

It gives a whole new meaning to the concept of fast food. I think of the couple joylessly eating pasties on the bench in the centre of town.

Tamworth's council is doing what it can to try to help people become more active. In 2010, it installed free outdoor gym equipment in the castle grounds and later in two other parks, Wigginton and Dosthill. It has built tennis courts and an outdoor skate park, instituted cycle hire and organised a sports festival to coincide with the arrival of the Olympic torch in 2012. It started outdoor Zumba classes. There are now about 15 council-run exercise and fitness classes a week, including Nordic walking. It invested £17,000 in free swimming lessons at a local pool and subsidised entry to the SnowDome's swimming pool.

Its efforts have achieved results. In 2009 just over 9,000 adults in Tamworth were taking part in sport, but by 2011, this had risen to 11,000. With a population of 76,000, however, there is still a way to go. It is, said Rob Barnes, 'a really good community leisure offer' but they need to change people's thinking if more are to use it. 'They have a perception that it is normal to be overweight, it is normal not to exercise and normal to smoke.'

Councillor Oates is concerned at how far things have gone. 'It's not just elderly but overweight people using mobility scooters,' he said. He recently saw four men of about his age with walking sticks. 'I thought, when did walking sticks become fashionable?' And then he realised these were overweight people who needed them to be able to get around.

'We're almost on the verge of a lost generation – obese parents who aren't recognising that their children are obese. Getting parents to recognise that is quite tricky,' he said.

But the efforts to combat the problem continue. GPs can now refer people with health problems caused by their weight to exercise classes run by the council. More than 2,400 were referred in 2011 and 2012. And it's not just about physical exercise. An eight-strong team of advisers give motivation and lifestyle support. The council says the outcomes are good and that 69 per cent of clients achieve part or all of the lifestyle changes they aim for.

In the castle grounds is a gym, crowded with exercise bikes and treadmills and the odd rowing machine.

It looks like a large hut – nothing in common with the glossy, plate-glass establishments blasting rhythmic music frequented by the young and aspirational professionals of our major cities. 'There are no mirrors and no Lycra,' said Karen Moss, the council's community sports manager. The people who attend this gym have no desire to ogle themselves or anybody else.

Squeeze into the room, without falling over the machines, and there are around 15 men, all past middle age, feet pounding on the moving belts, legs pumping the pedals. The only sounds are the thumps of serious physical exertion. They wear shorts and vests and come in various sizes of stout. All have the best possible motivation to get fitter. This is the cardiac rehabilitation group, referred to the gym because none of them wants another heart attack.

'I died twice,' said Stan Richardson, slightly short of breath from cycling. 'I was at the bowls club when I collapsed with a heart attack.' He had one and then another, three months later.

'I was all right until I packed in smoking,' he said. Then the retired van driver and delivery man put on weight until eventually he was over 100kg (16 stone).

Now, he says, after the heart attacks and the nutritional advice he has been given, he doesn't eat red meat or bacon but only chicken and fish. He admits to crisps, but 'only two to three bags a week – not every day,' he said. He is still a big man but, he says, 'It's muscle weight, not fat – that's why I'm overweight now.' Christmas was a problem, though. 'I had two weeks off [from the gym] and that buggered me. I started from scratch again.'

But for all the exercise initiatives, subsidised swimming and gym provision on the NHS, and an increasingly joined-up approach to public health which involves conversations and measures involving the education, environment and housing departments, the council is at a bit of a loss when it comes to tackling people's eating habits. What people eat has traditionally been their own business. The council has hardly been involved, beyond sorting things out when the building of new supermarkets looks likely to cause traffic jams.

It is the same in the north-east, where Gateshead shares the highest adult obesity rate in England with Tamworth, even though there are marked differences between the two towns which testify to how complex the causes of obesity really are and what a universal problem it is. An obvious issue is greater deprivation. As Carole Wood, Gateshead's director of public health, said, 'It is cultural, social and economic – and the economic factors are quite stark in Gateshead.'

But if you were going to put your finger on a single additional aggravation in Gateshead, it would probably be fish and chips. It's a way of life on the north-east coast. And it's a way to shorten life too. This is battered and deep-fried fish and chips as it used to be when it was key to feeding a hungry trawlerman who shortly had to go back out to sea and needed all the energy he could get to survive the coming storms – hot, substantial and cooked in beef dripping. These days the biggest enterprise in Gateshead is the

MetroCentre, which boasts of being the largest shopping mall in Europe, while the heavy industry of the Team Valley has largely given way to office-based businesses and retail.

But Gateshead folk have not all adopted a lighter diet to match the lighter physical workload. There has been no substitution of grilled fish with salad for fish and chips or pie and chips. Indeed, the chippies seem to be on the increase. 'We seem to be going through a proliferation of hot food takeaways. It is a feature of some of our communities,' said Wood. And do not be deceived by the healthy nature of fish. This is, says Wood, 'very high-fat fried food. I don't think we have one fish and chip shop or hot takeaway shop that would cook in vegetable oil rather than beef dripping.' And it's cheap. There are places where the density of takeaways leads to such competition that you can buy fish and chips for £1, she said.

Even if they want to eat more healthily, it may be hard for some families to find shops where they can buy fresh food to cook for themselves from scratch, rather than resorting to convenience meals in tins and packets in between takeaways. 'We are looking at doing a bit more study of this. In certain parts of Gateshead, unless you have a car it is much harder to access healthy food,' she said.

The council has been pondering whether it can restrict the numbers of takeaways or their positioning close to schools. Some other local authorities in the country have tried to take that road. But it's hard, she says. These are not the big food chains like McDonald's and Burger King that sign up to the government's Responsibility Deal, promising to cut the fat or salt content or list the calories of the meals they sell. These are small local businesses – and so they have an important role in the local economy. 'On the one hand, there is an economic issue around these small businesses setting up, but the sort of food being produced is cheap and high calorie and very high in saturated fat and salt, so there are also issues around people having access to that type of food in ever-growing amounts,' said Wood. The council has to weigh jobs against health.

Gateshead, on the south bank of the Tyne opposite Newcastle, has invested in the arts and culture. It is now famous for its pedestrian Millennium Bridge, which curves in a shining arch high over the river, and the huge Antony Gormley sculpture, the Angel of the North, whose 54-metre wingspan is visible from the A1. Its young people do far better at GCSE level than those in Tamworth – in 2009/10, 84.5 per cent got at least five A*–C grades.

But if these high educational standards and exposure to arts and culture are going to have an impact in helping the next generation rethink their lifestyles, it has not happened yet. And it is hard for anyone – young or old – to break with the social and cultural norms of their community. That goes for drinking too. Alcohol, said Wood, may also be an issue in Gateshead's obesity epidemic. Not only is it high in calories – 200 in a pint of Newcastle Brown – but alcohol also actually slows the body's ability to burn fat. In Gateshead, 44.5 per cent of men say they binge drink once a week or more, compared to 24.7 per cent in England as a whole, while 21.3 per cent of women in Gateshead admit to binge drinking compared to 15.4 per cent nationally. Gateshead residents also heavily exceed the safe weekly drinking limits.[3]

Lack of exercise may be less of a factor in Gateshead than in Tamworth. For those who want to resist the draw of videos and computer games and get off the sofa, the council has put in extensive cycle routes and bike parking, while for the summer, there are fabulous beaches. And, Wood points out, there are plenty of people in Gateshead who cannot afford to run a car and must walk and take public transport everywhere.

Gateshead council takes the view that obesity is an issue it must engage with – that it is not just a matter of personal responsibility. Besides, it can see the financial advantage in doing what it can. Excess weight and obesity cost the local NHS £64.3 million in 2010. By 2015, it estimated, that will be £68.7 million.

But both Tamworth and Gateshead say their options are limited. Wood in Gateshead talks about initiatives to teach cooking skills and encourage the older generation to pass down recipes to younger people – an inter-generational exchange that was once normal but has died out all over the country as people move away from their family homes and life speeds up.

Nor does the local authority have any control over food labelling or whether local stores stock fresh fruit or just high-fat, high-salt, high-sugar processed food and sweets. Today we eat 25 times more confectionery and drink 30 times more soft drinks than we did in the 1950s. These things are universally available, and what used to be a newsagent in Tamworth is now wall-to-wall packets of sweets, gums and chocolate bars of every imaginable variety, but almost all in extra-large sizes and usually on two-for-one offers.

Both Gateshead and Tamworth think that they need help from central government to tackle such a pervasive social, cultural and economic problem. 'I have never felt it [obesity] has been properly taken up,' said Wood. 'I think it needs clear leadership at the national level. With any public health programme, especially one as complex as [the one required to tackle] obesity, you need clear leadership and it has to be multi-faceted.' Obesity is an issue for schools, education, transport, employment and environment as well as health, she says.

In Tamworth, just before I left and hungry after having skipped lunch, I went into Costa Coffee for a sandwich. Around half to a third of the people there were visibly overweight, including a young mother at the table next to me. She had a sandwich and a large latte, her partner had a large cappuccino and on the table was a cup of whipped cream as well – into which they dipped the dummy of the toddler beside them, strapped in her pushchair. When she had sucked off the cream, she shouted for more and they took it in turns to give her more … and more … and more. Maybe it was because I had been pondering for so long why one town should have more obesity than another, but I admit to being shocked. What made this couple give their two-year-old thick, sweet cream, rather than milk or even water? Were they not worried that the taste she was developing for it would set her up for obesity in later life? I wanted to ask them, but of course thought better of it. Our culture says we do not interfere. What we eat – and give our children to eat – is our own responsibility, most would say.

But others would argue that in Tamworth, in Gateshead and everywhere else in Britain and around the world, our convenient, fast-paced, car-dominated society, our free-market embrace of the cheap processed food and soft drinks industry and the cultural norms of the 'have it all' society, which has come to mean 'eat it all' as well, appear to be working against anyone who would like to maintain a healthy weight. If too many people are obese in Tamworth and Gateshead, do we dare to say it is their fault?

5

SO WHERE'S THE HARM?

We don't think of weight as a health issue, but as an image issue. We think it's something for gossip magazines, not medical textbooks and doctor's waiting rooms. As a direct result, politicians are able to sideline our growing weight problems and do nothing to prevent obesity getting worse. Who is going to call them to account? Obesity is not a voting issue.

And there are other consequences. Many people with weight issues feel stigmatised and unfairly treated because we judge them on their appearance. Some are angry and believe it's all just about prejudice and an obsession with supermodels – a sick culture which sees stick-thin skinny catwalk models as desirably shaped. Meanwhile there is wrangling between the scientists over the extent of the damage our junk-food habit is causing us, instead of the unambiguous clarity we need.

In 2013, a huge row broke out when Katherine Flegal published a paper showing that overweight and mildly obese people did not die any sooner than anyone else.

Flegal was not trying to slaughter sacred cows. It's not generally what US government employees do. She is an epidemiologist. She believes in numbers. But her paper in the *Journal of the American Medical Association*, one of the leading medical journals in the world, triggered a storm of fury and anxiety.

Flegal, who works for the National Center for Health Statistics of the Centers for Disease Control and Prevention in Maryland, is a major figure in obesity research – one of those who started the ball rolling. Back in 1994, she was one of the first to alert the USA to its soaring obesity rates, when she and colleagues published the first of a series of studies based on government data. These made people sit up and realise what was happening and consider not only the impact on people's health but also how much it was going to cost health services to care for them. Academics began to study obesity as an issue, campaigning groups were set up, public health experts became involved. The perceived problems associated with being overweight, in short, were no longer about body image and who could fit into a size zero dress. They moved out of the women's magazines and became a major medical issue, troubling politicians too. Funding started to flow into the field and people began building expertise and careers.

But then two papers by Flegal and colleagues – a smaller one in 2005 and then the big review of all the worthwhile scientific studies that the team could lay their hands on in 2013 – appeared to threaten all that and strengthen the hand of critics who said that politicians and scientists alike should not interfere and that our weight is our own responsibility. Flegal and colleagues' work was taken as evidence that the problem had been massively overblown. Why all the fuss if people do not die of mild obesity after all? Maybe being fat doesn't actually harm you all that much.

The January 2013 paper pooled the results of 97 studies of weight and mortality, which in total had data on 2.88 million adults, among whom there were more than 270,000 deaths.

If you looked at all those who were obese together, then yes, they did die earlier than people of normal weight (classified as a BMI of 18.5 to 25). But the mildly obese, with a BMI of 30 to 35, were no more likely to suffer an early death than people of normal weight. And those who were classified as overweight, with a BMI of 25 to 30, actually had longer lives. Somehow, having a few extra pounds was protective.

Apple carts were overturned – and indeed their contents slung at Flegal's head. Other scientists – some of them worried that an erroneously dangerous message that obesity is harmless would get out – weighed in with heavy boots. The most damning line came from Dr Walter Willett of the Harvard School of Public Health, who had also dismissed the 2005 paper. 'This study is really a pile of rubbish, and no one should waste their time reading it,' he said on National Public Radio.

Who is to say, he asked, that the thin people in this paper, who died early, were healthy thin people? Flegal's sums did not take account of those who are thin because they are ill – and therefore more likely to die. And anyway, focusing just on deaths ignores the massively important issue of chronic disease like diabetes and heart trouble, which can wreck your quality of life. Even if you don't die of it, he was saying, you could be facing a lifetime of unnecessary suffering from disease. 'We have a huge amount of other literature showing that people who gain weight or are over-weight have increased risk of diabetes, heart disease, stroke, many cancers and many other conditions,' Willett said.

Across the Atlantic, Professor John Wass, vice-president of the Royal College of Physicians, also went on the offen-sive. 'Have you ever seen a 100-year-old human being who is overweight? The answer is you probably haven't,' he said. 'Huge pieces of evidence go against this. Countless other studies point in the other direction.'

Flegal, speaking on NPR after the deluge, was rueful. 'Our article got called rubbish and ludicrous … so it really opens you to lots of criticism. I discovered much to my sorrow that this is kind of a flashpoint for people.'

The problem is that science is anything but black and white. Contrary to what a lot of people think, it does not deliver conclusive answers – or only to the most simple of questions. The statistics on the computer screen may be correct, but the tricky part is figuring out what they mean in the real world.

Flegal and her fellow authors said as much in the paper, offering a number of possible explanations for what they had found. Why do people who are a bit overweight live longer than those whose weight is normal? Well, maybe carrying too many pounds can cause you to get ill – but once you are sick, perhaps they may help you recover more quickly than somebody who is thin. Thin is not always healthy or robust. People with cancer get emaciated and weak. Your body may cope better if you have more flesh to start with.

Or maybe, they suggested, health problems get picked up sooner if you are heavier. Doctors and nurses suspect you may have health problems. Excess weight, like high blood pressure, is a flashing light for them. So heavier people may get offered screening for heart problems or diabetes and so get earlier treatment, which gives them a better chance of recovery.

But this sort of nuanced reasoning in the fine print towards the end of the paper wasn't going to satisfy those of Flegal's critics who felt the headline message was plain dangerous. Obesity, they were saying, is not OK and it is irresponsible to suggest there is any way it might be. The debate was heated and the messenger became a target for shooting practice. In fact, there are points on both sides, but obesity is such a sensitive issue that nobody seemed able to discuss it without rancour.

Quite a few of Flegal's critics took the opportunity to rubbish the basic obesity measurement used in almost all research – the body mass index, or BMI. It was far from the first time. There has long been a major argument over how you can measure obesity at all.

Basically, BMI is a flawed measure – and that is putting it a lot more politely than its critics. Most people agree it isn't perfect, but they come back to it every time for two reasons:

firstly, it's the measure that anybody anywhere can work out, because the only information you need to collect are people's weight and height. Secondly, because everybody else uses it, there is data already available that scientists can reasonably use to compare obesity in different communities around the world. So the academics and public health experts cling to it.

But BMI was never intended to be the personal weight test it has become – almost as universally used in the doctor's surgery as our pulse or blood-pressure reading. It was invented by Adolphe Quetelet, a multi-talented Belgian who lived in the 1800s. He was a mathematician, astronomer, statistician and sociologist and one of the first to introduce probability and statistics to the social sciences. He wanted to establish patterns and work out underlying probabilities in crime, marriage and suicide rates.

So Quetelet's index was a population measure and as such, BMI is a simple and useful tool. BMI these days is calculated as a person's mass (or weight) in kilograms divided by their height in metres squared. Those figures are readily available for populations in developed countries, making it easy to get a handle on the sort of numbers who are overweight, underweight and obese. That's good for health ministers who want to know how much they are probably going to have to spend on diabetes in 30 years' time. But it's a rough and ready reckoning when it comes to individuals. Bodybuilders, athletes and people in the military with hard-packed muscles can end up with the same high BMI as somebody with a lot of excess flab. On a weighing machine, it is all just extra kilos or pounds. And the basic calculation takes no account of your age, sex or race – although a lot of the websites offering it will factor at least age and sex in when giving you a verdict.

Willett, Flegal's most ferocious critic, was one of those who argued that it was wrong to use BMI to figure out how overweight people were without taking into account their general state of fitness and health. Others joined him. A top Canadian obesity expert, Dr Arya Sharma, a professor at Alberta University, argued the BMI's credibility was already shot to pieces and hoped it would now be permanently laid to rest. In his blog he pointed out that he and his team had recently published their own analysis of US data in the *Canadian Medical Association Journal*. They found, he said, that 'when it comes to mortality, what matters is how "sick" you are and not how "big" you are. If you have a weight-related health problem … you die, if not, you don't – end of story!

'As we outline in our paper, not only would BMI overestimate health problems in millions of US citizens, it would also completely miss about 25 million Americans, who do have weight-related health issues, despite falling well below the BMI 30 obesity range.

'Perhaps, after this paper, we can finally lay BMI to rest and stop trying to predict people's health with just scales and measuring tapes.

'Hopefully, the only landmark that this paper leaves behind is a tombstone – BMI – RIP!'[1]

To get over the failings of BMI, doctors are increasingly measuring waistlines. It isn't fat all over which matters – it is fat around the middle. Pear-shaped people with weight on their hips have less to worry about. It is apple-shaped people who may be in trouble. Waist measurement will give you an idea of how much visceral or internal fat you have – that white stuff that shows up so dramatically on an MRI scan. Hip and thigh fat is designed to store energy. The really serious problem is not the subcutaneous fat just under your skin that makes you look plump, but the fat you cannot see that is wrapped around your internal organs – around your liver, your heart or your pancreas.

Jean-Pierre Després, a Canadian doctor who poses for pictures outside the Laval University in Québec, where he is director of cardiology research, with a pair of running shoes and a tape measure, travels the world advocating waist measurement over BMI to anybody who will listen. 'We can no longer define obesity on the basis of excess body weight,' he told me. 'If you judge only by BMI, there are some obese people who are perfectly healthy, while others of normal weight have medical problems you would not suspect.'

Després is scientific director of an organisation which labours under the imponderable title of the International Chair on Cardiometabolic Risk – no doubt because it is primarily focused on persuading doctors to get out the tape measure it has as its logo rather than talking to the public. Its website is well titled – myhealthywaist.org – but apart from some useful diagrams on exactly where to put the tape, it is science heavy. Yet the bottom line is almost incredibly simple – a waist measuring more than 80cm in a European or North American woman or 94cm in a man means you have stores of dangerous abdominal or visceral fat that put you at increased risk of diabetes and other disease. A waistline of 108cm in a man or 88cm in a woman is a major risk factor. (The figures are slightly different for people of Chinese, Japanese and South Asian origin, while sub-Saharan African, Latin Americans and Arabic populations are advised to use the European numbers until more data is available.)

'The bad news is that inner fat is bad for you,' said Després. 'The good news is that inner fat is very susceptible to lifestyle changes. There is plenty of data to show that better diet and more exercise can reduce it.' Després sees both the problem and the solution in relatively simple terms. He is an exercise enthusiast – he studied the effects of exercise on the body before taking a medical degree. Get moving, he says. We should all be physically active for 150 minutes a week, he says. It would do us all good – it's the sedentary lifestyle that is the killer. 'Exercise is cardio-protective and also a powerful tool to mobilise the fat around your heart and liver.' (Nonetheless he does also suggest we cut the sugar and salt levels in our diet and stay off the sweetened soft drinks. 'You can't ban them, but the population should be aware that cans of pop are useless to your system. These pleasure drinks are not the way we should hydrate ourselves,' he said.)

Després and his colleagues believe waist measurement provides a more meaningful target for people trying to lose weight. 'If you drop your waistline by 4cm, you can reduce your risk of developing type 2 diabetes by 60 per cent,' he said. It doesn't mean you lose pounds necessarily because you could have more muscle, but some of the internal fat will have been dispersed.

But while the academics and the scientists are throwing eggs at each other, each trying to prove the other has got it wrong, millions of people who think they may have a problem or *know* they have a problem, because they labour to climb the stairs or are on hefty medication to keep their blood pressure down, are left in confusion and without help. Academic wrangling over the size and scale of the problem allows the food and drink industry to do business as usual and the politicians to smile, albeit uneasily, from the sidelines. And this lack of clarity allows the ignorant attitudes of the nastier and more unfeeling members of society towards the overweight to go unchallenged. Fat kids are bullied in the playground. Fat women are jeered and mocked. Fat men are the butt of jokes – although far less likely to suffer unpleasantness than women, who are expected to be on a perpetual diet if they fail to have a catwalk supermodel figure.

A significant number of overweight and obese people feel they have always been stigmatised for their size and are now being oppressed by scientists, doctors and the media, who talk of an epidemic and a threat to the world's healthcare systems and economies.

The 'war on obesity', they feel, has become a war on fat people. Many have been on countless diets that have not worked, but despite their efforts to lose weight they encounter discrimination, disbelief and derision. They feel they are being blamed for being a size and shape that our culture does not admire and for burdening the health service. Fat activism has grown up to champion the legions of heavy people who feel rejected and stigmatised. The fat acceptance movement Health At Every Size (HAES) is part of this development, advocating that it is not weight or your appearance that matters, but your fitness and overall health.

Angela Meadows, a doctoral researcher at Birmingham University's department of psychology, organised the first ever weight stigma conference in the UK in May 2013. She has a BMI of 40 and a dress size of 20 and, she says – so what?

'Statistically speaking, people who are fit have very, very similar and good health outcomes regardless of their weight – even if they are overweight, even if they are obese – very similar to people of normal weight. Even if they are obese they do better than people who are thin and aren't fit,' she said.

The conference was a packed and passionate gathering in a seminar room of the university, which got heated in every sense. There were academics, students and health professionals, most of them committed, angry at the stigmatisation of people who are overweight, and it felt more like a rally than a debating chamber – a rare chance for an oppressed and angry group to let off steam. Why is it, asked one, that when glamorous, thin, sexually attractive actresses pretend to be fat, as Monica did in *Friends*, they are portrayed as stupid, clumsy nerds? 'When she gets into the fat suit, her whole personality changes. She becomes this clumsy, silly, stupid person – and that's what women are afraid of! They are afraid of risking their social status.'

Meadows argues that a lot of the health problems that fat people (the HAES movement has reclaimed the F-word, she says) suffer are not to do with the weight they carry, but are in fact the result of the massive stigma they experience, which leads to self-loathing and poor mental and physical health.

She told me appalling tales of the daily stress and pressure that fat people are under: 'People mooing at them on the street, people throwing eggs at them when they are exercising.' She even described one occasion when an overweight friend was at the supermarket and a fellow shopper – somebody she did not know – actually reached into her trolley and removed a packet of biscuits, insisting she did not need them.

'People are being asked to leave shops because they are not projecting the right image for the customers they want to attract. They say, we don't want you in here – please don't stand in front of the shop either. It is not just the stigma itself but [also] the expectation that people are going to treat you like this every time you step outside your front door that massively impacts on people's lives,' she said.

So fat people don't go out. They stay at home and hide from the mob. 'They tend not to join a gym, not to go out with their friends for a meal because they don't want to be seen eating in public. They don't travel, they don't fly, they don't take a job that requires them to fly because they're worried about people being mean to them and fitting into seats that are too narrow for them,' she said.

'These kind of things massively, massively impact on people's lives and relationships ... they become drug addicts, commit suicide,[2] become an alcoholic. It really is quite horrifying and it is not just the blatant stuff, like people throwing eggs at you. It really is the everyday fear that people are looking down on you and devaluing you.'

The Yale Rudd Center for Food Policy and Obesity has pulled together the evidence on stigma in the US, where the problem has been most researched.[3] Fat people are less likely to get good grades in school – they are thought stupid – and less likely to get good jobs and promotions, Meadows says. They are mocked and derided. 'And I think for the people who haven't discovered size acceptance yet, it's even worse because they believe it – they believe they deserve that because they are so disgusting and so fat. They think they must be a terrible burden and they deserve to be treated like that. That self-loathing, of course, has additional negative effects.'

Meadows was dieting and hating herself from the age of 12 or 13, she said. She talks of suffering more than two decades of misery and hurt before, while studying biomedical science and on her way to a Masters in weight management and a qualification as a physical trainer, she discovered what she calls the fitness/fatness data. She was shocked and curious, she says – and now she says she has got her life back.

'For me, I know a certain number of people will think I'm worthless because I'm fat but I don't believe it. I don't have that internalisation. I just think it's their problem.'

Like racial discrimination and homophobia, the sort of prejudice and denigration and the resulting self-loathing that fat people endure have serious effects on their health, she says. She believes it is this that is increasing their risk of high blood pressure, heart disease and diabetes – not the fat. She cites a study from Columbia University in New York that showed the more unhappy people were with their weight, the more unhealthy they were likely to be.[4] 'In other words, feeling bad about themselves actually makes them sicker,' she said. And dieting makes people worse. They lose some pounds over a couple of months and then put it all back on – and more. The body fears starvation and actively works to minimise weight loss. The more you diet, the more you fail and the more miserable you feel about yourself.

Years of scorn, rejection and yo-yo dieting have made radicals of some of the fat-acceptance movement members, angry at their treatment and suggestions from the thin that they don't try. Meadows does not dispute the link between heart disease and diabetes and extreme weight in people who are not fit. But, she says, look at people's health – don't make assumptions from the scales.

'HAES doesn't say you can be healthy at any size,' she says. 'It doesn't say that the 800-lb man sitting in his house is healthy – it says that whatever your weight is, wherever you are starting from, if you want to improve your health, start doing healthy things, start taking care of yourself, start trying to move, even if it is a little bit, start nourishing your body, and that is your best shot at improving your health.'

What she and others most want is better understanding. She writes letters to the newspapers complaining of pictures of what she calls 'headless fatties' – the photo of a bulging stomach with no face attached, which is invariably used to illustrate obesity stories. You argue in vain with her that it seems intrusive to use people's faces. To her, the pictures are further stigmatisation of fat as something revolting and likely to increase the prejudices of readers.

There is no doubt that some fat people have suffered severely from the jibes and prejudice of others around them – particularly those like Meadows who encountered stigma decades ago as children. But something fundamental has happened which must surely change that. Overweight people are not a minority. Nearly two-thirds of us are over-weight or obese. Research also shows that obesity runs in communities – if your close circle of friends is fat, it is more likely you will be too. That means there is a good chance the people you care about and socialise with will look like you. They are not going to call you rude names in the street or confiscate your biscuits in the supermarket.

Jane Wardle, professor of psychology at the health behaviour research centre of University College London, does not believe that obese and overweight people are unhappier today than thin ones. She has a graph to show it in a large group of women over the age of 50. They are divided up into six groups by weight, from underweight to normal weight to severely obese. When they were questioned in detail about their 'life satisfaction', all six groups of women scored almost exactly the same.

Stigma, she says, has been studied more in other areas of life than in obesity, but on the whole it appears, she says, that it does not always affect self-esteem in the way you might expect. 'The psychologists who write about it, interestingly, say that many of us in various different ways have to cope with the slings and arrows of our fellow citizens for one thing or another and part of what might build self-confidence is learning to feel OK about yourself even if everybody is not necessarily telling you that you are OK.

'I have treated lots of overweight and obese people and got quite a few of them as friends. I have no doubt that they are treated unreasonably and unfairly in various different ways but this doesn't actually seem to be, for most of the time and for most people, worse than just a difficult thing [one has] to live with, like having your father die or getting old. People's self-esteem and wellbeing aren't as fragile as that.'

Obesity was sometimes treated as a psychological disease in the 1950s, Wardle says, when it was pretty rare, affecting maybe 6 or 7 per cent of the population. 'People would quite often be sent to psychoanalysts – not that anyone ever did any studies that showed this made any difference. That was the sort of thinking – that surely if you can exert willpower than you wouldn't need to be fat, ergo you've got a shortage of willpower, therefore probably some kind of psychological support would help you engage this willpower.' But when large studies started to be done, nobody could find any real link between psychopathology and weight.

These days, she says, the evidence does show that people who go for obesity treatment appear more depressed – but it's possible the depression, triggered by other things in their life, is driving them to the doctor, because they think the solution to how they feel is to get a grip on their weight problem.

But most obese people do not arrive at the doctor's door because they feel unhappy. Most get there because they have begun to experience serious physical problems related to their weight. Their knees are painful because their joints are under too much pressure. They are tired, drowsy and suffering from extreme thirst with the early symptoms of diabetes. Or they have a heart attack.

The numbers arriving in hospital are dismaying front-line doctors. Many diabetes specialists and heart disease experts are overwhelmed by the number of patients they are seeing who are substantially overweight and sick. And these doctors are increasingly willing to enter the political fray. There is a huge body of doctors and public health experts who now say obesity is claiming lives and destroying health and that it will only get worse, as the processed food and drink industry expands into every corner of the globe. This is not about stigmatising fat people – and has nothing at all to do with body image, fashion magazine diet tips or gossip about celebrity cellulite.

The Global Burden of Disease study, a mammoth affair mapping the harm from every health threat known to man conducted by the Institute of Health Metrics and Evaluation at the University of Washington in Seattle, crunched the global numbers in 2012 and came up with a startling finding. For the first time, they said in their series published by the *Lancet* medical journal, obesity was harming more people in the world than under-nutrition. More people are dangerously fat than starving. According to Philip James of IASO, in his chapter in the *Oxford Textbook of Public Health*, high BMI is 'a rapidly escalating major public health problem affecting most countries in the world' and 'the fastest-growing risk factor for global health'. The WHO estimates that approximately 1.46 billion people around the world are overweight and 502 million of these are obese. It's a massive global health problem.

What will it do to you? Putting on too much weight can cause high blood pressure, raised cholesterol levels in your blood and raised glucose levels – or if you already suffer in that way, it can make them worse. Those conditions can lead to life-shortening or life-ruining diseases.

The illnesses that overweight people are most likely to suffer are diabetes, gallbladder disease, breathlessness and sleep apnoea. Heart disease, stroke, high blood pressure, osteoarthritis and gout are moderately likely. There is an increased risk of breast cancer (after the age of 50), bowel, kidney and pancreatic cancer, fertility problems, low back pain and early dementia. There is also a raised risk that the baby of an obese woman will suffer damage in the womb.

Many of these illnesses carry severe consequences. Cardiovascular disease – heart disease and stroke – is one of the main causes of premature death (defined as before the age of 75). In the UK, there were 42,000 premature deaths in 2011.

The inexorable rise of obesity and related diseases has filled medics with alarm and, increasingly, anger, as politicians have taken little or no action. The tide of concern eventually led to the United Nations convening the first ever high-level meeting on 'non-communicable diseases' – an infinitely forgettable and uninformative blanket term for everything that is not infectious. They are talking about the chronic diseases that have their origins in our modern lifestyles: cancer, heart disease, stroke, diabetes and lung conditions. All are caused or worsened by obesity.

In a special issue on obesity in 2011, just ahead of the UN summit, an international group of concerned doctors led by Boyd Swinburn from Melbourne, Australia wrote one of a series of papers for the *Lancet* medical journal, laying it on the line. 'Governments have largely abdicated responsibility for obesity, leaving this to the individual NGOs and the private sector,' they said.

In the medical community, obesity is becoming a radicalising issue, just as HIV was in the years before there were drugs to stop people dying. In the US and the UK, doctors are increasingly going public and becoming more pointedly critical of the politicians. Too little is being done, they say. And, they add, too often people are being blamed for their weight, as an excuse for those in power to do nothing to help them.

In January 2013, the Royal College of Physicians in the UK published a report calling for more action to prevent obesity and more resources for doctors to deal with the consequences. NHS services are 'extremely patchy', said the report. 'Obesity is an increasing and costly public health problem which is not being addressed by current services or policy.' Professor John Wass, chair of the working party that wrote the report and academic vice-president of the RCP, said: 'Britain is getting bigger and whilst we try to prevent the increase in obesity, we must also prepare the NHS for the influx of patients presenting with severe complex obesity. A patient may arrive at my hospital with coronary heart disease, but if the root cause of their condition is obesity, we must be equipped to deal with that root cause.'

Desperate for action, Wass told me that we ought to have somebody in the public eye to lead the social change that is needed to combat obesity to whom everybody would listen, alongside a seasoned government operator who could make diverse departments like health, education, transport and planning work together. For the former, he had in mind the British equivalent of Michelle Obama – royalty.

'Let us say – real pie in the sky – we had a member of the royal family leading with a crossbench peer who had experience across departments of government. We'd be one of the countries that could solve the problem first on the planet,' he said. 'We could get a lot achieved by enthusiasm and efficiency. In the medical profession there is a burning desire to get the services in place.'

The UK's public health doctors are on board – how could they not be? It is their job to identify and tackle the malign influences around us that damage our health, from poor sanitation in Victorian times, to cigarettes, alcohol and now our calorific diet and sedentary lives. Lindsey Davies, president of the Faculty of Public Health, is outspoken on the subject. In an important statement, she backed the call for cross-departmental action from the government – and slammed politicians for blaming people for their weight.

'Obesity is not only caused by how much we each eat or drink: if tackling it were as simple as telling people to eat less and move more, we would have solved it by now,' she said.

'Our chances of being obese are also affected by factors like whether we have easy access to affordable fruit, veg and other healthy foods, and if it is safe to let our kids play outside. That's why if governments focus on personal choice alone it is at best a red herring and at worst a dere-liction of duty for everyone's health.'

Personal choice is a red herring and governments must act. That shows the real gulf between doctors and the politi-cians – who persist in seeing the processed food industry as an economic motor and not a threat to the nation's health. Just a month after that broadside, a second report from the UK's doctors appeared. The Academy of Medical Royal Colleges, which spans all the disciplines, launched an even more overtly political tome.

'We are grappling with one of the biggest threats to public health in the 21st century,' they argued. They called for £100 million to be invested in weight-reduction programmes in each of the four countries of the UK, to match anti-smoking efforts. More remarkably, their report laid into the food and drink industry, called for a ban on junk-food advertising to children on TV and a sugary drinks tax of at least 20 per cent. This, for doctors, was as political as they get.

Terence Stephenson, Academy president and a paediatrician, was the driving force behind the report. He says there are clear parallels between the behaviour of the food industry and that of the tobacco industry of old. The food and drink industry now 'rubbish the evidence whenever they can, question it, lobby against it', he told me.

'There are two things where they deviate from the tobacco industry. One is they say that nobody has to smoke cigarettes, whereas everybody has to eat. So they kind of use that as one of their things – eating is a healthy thing,' he said.

'The second thing is, they say, well, everybody in the world who eats a balanced diet will get perhaps a third of their calories or more from carbohydrates and this is true of six billion people across the globe, so what's your problem? But most of those six billion aren't eating highly refined sugars, they're not eating Crunchie bars and Coca-Cola. They're eating brown rice, they're eating their crops, they are subsistence farming. Calories are not readily available in huge amounts and you don't get this rapid kick in your blood sugar to the same extent.'

He believes it is time for legislation in the shape of a tax on sweet drinks. Government has to help us do what is best for us. Human nature is too frail and the forces ranked against us too great. 'In theory, of course, we should all be better people,' he told me. 'We should be more upright, better behaved – but we tax lots of things because of human nature. Our spirits are willing but the flesh is weak, as my mother would have said. We tax alcohol, we tax cigarettes – for that matter, we tax petrol – so there are lots of things where the free market is recognised not necessarily to work for the benefit of people. We don't tax illicit drugs, we actually ban them. So as a civilised society, we don't actually allow a free market to operate. That may seem extreme, but in a sense sugar is probably killing more people now than alcohol, I guess – or it must be getting very close.'

That summer, in June 2013, the American Medical Association meeting in Chicago voted to recognise obesity as a disease. Doctors in the United States also felt that a watershed had been reached and more needed to be done. 'Recognising obesity as a disease will help change the way the medical community tackles this complex issue that affects approximately one in three Americans,' said AMA board member Patrice Harris in a statement. 'The AMA is committed to improving health outcomes and is working to reduce the incidence of cardiovascular disease and type 2 diabetes, which are often linked to obesity.' That overtly political decision could potentially change things radically for obese people in America, according to the Obesity Action Coalition, which represents patients. They can no longer be dismissed as weak or foolish people who indulge in an ill-advised lifestyle and hold the remedy in their own hands – they have a health problem that doctors must help them address.

Doctors are getting political because most of them feel helpless to stop the epidemic in its tracks. They don't have a vaccine. Those in primary care are in a position to talk to patients who arrive with bad knees and breathlessness about their weight – but many of them do not. The stigma is such that some doctors fear they will cause anger or distress. They don't have the language. Obese is a hard word and fat is a rude one. Others know from experience that losing weight is incredibly difficult and all they have to offer is a diet sheet and possibly gym membership. And the mindset most of them enter into from medical school is that their job is to treat people who are sick. Few feel comfortable dishing out lifestyle advice.

Instead, doctors are encouraged by NICE to hand out statins, cheap cholesterol-lowering drugs, to all those who have more than a 10 per cent risk of developing heart disease. Some 7 million people are now taking them in the UK, but although the drugs are pretty safe, there are side-effects and they are no substitute for lifestyle changes. They reduce the chances of a heart attack or stroke (but not by very much) and the drug company-funded studies have not shown they cut the risk of a premature death.[5]

That is why it is the specialists who are making the running. They see people arriving in droves with preventable illness. Some of them, according to psychologist Professor Jane Ogden, who sees them in her clinics in Surrey, are in great distress about their weight. One woman said about her daughter, 'My kid came out of school and she was so upset because they'd really been on at her all day and she said, "Why can't you just be skinny like everybody else's mum?"' Ogden told the Birmingham stigma conference. Another said, 'I didn't feel like a person – I felt like some great blob wobbling around. I hated myself. I absolutely hated myself. I just thought I was worthless – no good to anyone. Often I felt like killing myself.'

Ogden reflected on how serious obesity had become. When she first started working in obesity, it was with people who were size 16 and thought they had a problem. 'Now I'm seeing people in wheelchairs who get stuck in the bath and can't wipe their own bottom and have a pretty grim time,' she said.

One of the main reasons for doctors' frustration is that there is so little treatment for obesity. Diets don't work in the long term for most people and nor do drugs. The one intervention that does make a dramatic difference is surgery to reduce the size of the stomach so that people just cannot eat so much at one sitting.

Sally Norton, bariatric surgeon with the North Bristol NHS Trust, is the last hope of the desperate. Adapting the human body on the operating table so that people can deal with the barrage of food signals around them in the modern world is a drastic measure, worthy of a dystopian novel. But it can be a life-saver.

Norton, like Ogden, sees the desperate cases – the people unable to walk and who find it hard to breathe, whose lives have been destroyed by their weight. Others have a BMI only just in the morbidly obese category, but there is every sign that they will have severe health problems if they continue as they are. 'There is something to be said for operating earlier rather than waiting for people to get in such a bad state,' she said. 'By the time you're in a wheelchair crippled with arthritis, we're less likely to get you back to work. We might improve your mobility and your reliance on carers but we want to get you back into work.'

This is not about supermodels and celebrities and size-zero bodies. There is nothing remotely cosmetic about it. The public perception that this surgery is about looking good and has anything in common with a nose job is completely awry. They have the wrong idea, she thinks, because private cosmetic clinics, some of them abroad, are selling weight-loss surgery along with boob jobs.

'They show [on their website] all these pictures of people who have lost lots of weight and looking glamorous. So we're fighting against that perception,' she told me.

'I think the message is becoming clearer, certainly among the general health profession. It's becoming clear that what we're doing is improving health, not just making people slimmer. But it's the message that we have to keep putting across.'

Surgery is the drastic option and it's only for the morbidly obese. This is not liposuction, which removes some of the fat below the skin but does nothing about the crucial and deadly visceral fat around the organs. Bariatric surgeons alter the stomach with which you were born, so that it will no longer function as nature intended. Most of it is removed or bypassed, so that only a small pouch remains and it becomes physically very difficult and unpleasant to eat more than tiny amounts.

It's not to be undertaken lightly. It's available on the NHS only to people above a BMI of 40 or those with a BMI of more than 35 who are suffering from obesity-related ill-health. And they must have tried for a long time to lose weight in other ways – through diets and drugs – before they will be accepted. Yet the public still judges them.

'There is still a lack of sympathy for these patients,' Norton told me. 'The perception is that they are just lazy and greedy and not doing much to help themselves, but actually the vast majority of the patients we see are desperately trying to sort themselves out. They've been on countless diets and we know conventional diets don't work.

'Quite frequently – about 25 per cent in some studies – they have got severe psychological issues. They might have very traumatic childhoods or past physical or mental abuse. All those issues shape how their behaviour has developed over the years and we have to tackle all of that, so we spend a lot of time going through those psychological issues and other health problems before we will consider weight-loss surgery.'

Bariatric surgery can transform lives. People can go out again. They can go back to work. It is not just cost-effective for the health service, reducing the numbers of hip replacements, knee replacements and treatment for all sorts of other physical ailments. It is also good for the economy.

But it is not as widely available as it should be. The problem is not the queue for the operating theatre, but a shortage of clinics where people can go for the long period of physical and psychological assessment and counselling that they need before they go under the knife.

Norton, on the council of the British Obesity and Metabolic Surgery Society, is working to get more people into the system. In Bristol, she and colleagues have been running clinics to assess and monitor patients for years. There's no question of anybody going straight to theatre. It is crucial that they have the help of psychologists, dieticians and doctors to try to lose weight in other ways first and prepare them for the serious change to their life that surgery will bring. But the NHS is playing catch-up. Not every area has what is called a tier 3 service – the assessment and monitoring clinics that are required before a patient can get surgery. Even in Bristol, the clinics Norton and her colleagues have been running have not yet had the official tier 3 stamp.

In some areas, you can be told you will be waiting for years. That sends some of the desperate into the arms of private clinics either in the UK or abroad. Norton says that is a real worry.

'I wouldn't be encouraging people to have surgery abroad because they can end up getting inappropriate surgery. There are people we wouldn't have dreamed of operating on because of psychological or other issues and they've gone abroad and had surgery and [then] the NHS has got a difficult problem to deal with,' she said.

'If somebody's got, for example, a history of bulimia – or one example was swallowing razor blades – that's not a good patient to put forward for a gastric band. If somebody like that came to us, we would obviously give them a lot of psychological counselling and treatment before we even contemplated surgery, but if they just go off abroad they can get it done the next day.'

People wrongly assume that if you have surgery, that's an end to it. You can no longer eat so much. If you try, you will quickly feel full and if you persist, you will probably vomit. But it's not a quick fix. People need a lot of help afterwards. Your diet has to change – you can eat some foods and not others. And you have to negotiate social occasions – what do you tell people who invite you round to dinner, when you will have to leave half the meal on the plate? There is also a danger you will still end up eating the wrong foods. If you are obsessed with sweets and cakes and puddings, how are you going to ensure you have room for vegetables and fruit and protein? Nobody should be left to cope with the difficult post-gastric band road alone. Some people need lifelong support. But clinics overseas cannot offer the aftercare people need and private clinics may charge more than people can afford. Norton sees the fallout as people return to the NHS with problems. Without the counselling and support they need, complications can set in. In the end, they develop a medical problem which the NHS will have to put right and that costs more in the long run.

There needs to be a more sympathetic approach to such people, she says. They should not be ignored by the NHS until such time as they develop more health problems. Australia, she says, gets better results from gastric-band surgery than the UK. 'Patients are seen more regularly, so they get counselling or dietetic support,' she said. Some people will need adjustments to their gastric band or occasionally a revision. 'It is a fairly minor operation if you catch it early enough, but if you don't get that support then small problems turn into big problems or people feel a bit left out on a limb or they just fall back into bad habits. And that's actually crazy, because that sort of support is cheap compared to surgery or managing the complications of being obese.'

People can lose half their weight after stomach surgery, but only if they have managed to make changes to the way they live. The stomach, says Norton, is a stretchable organ. It is very possible for people to regain all of the weight they lose and more.

We can't treat our way out of the obesity epidemic. Only in science fiction could we surgically alter most of the human race to cope with the junk-food explosion. Norton, dealing with the casualties on the battlefield, believes that so much more needs to be done to prevent them getting harmed in the first place. She admits she is completely overwhelmed by the problems she sees.

Norton is angry about the junk food that is pushed in our faces. She feels passionate about it, talking about the impossibility even of getting a healthy apple while on a night shift in the hospital because all the vending machines are full of chocolate bars. 'We're constantly fighting our surroundings and all the advertising. I feel so sorry for the younger generation who have such a struggle ahead to keep their weight under control in an environment like this. Just go into the local cinema where a large coke can be one third of your daily calorie requirement – let alone the popcorn – and it's clear they don't stand a chance.'

When I talk to her, she is in the middle of an email argument with the leading UK chain of health-food stores, Holland and Barrett, after pointing out to them that they had a big display of jellybeans in the middle of one of their shops. 'This is one of our major health-food retailers in the high street. What on earth is going on there if they are promoting that as a health food in the middle of their store? People will be walking in there and thinking jelly-beans are healthy when they are mostly sugar,' she said. Gourmet Jelly Beans – fruit cocktail flavours – are adver-tised also on the Holland and Barrett website. The first listed ingredient is sugar, followed by glucose syrup. Sugars make up 31g of every 40g tube.

Stopping people becoming overweight has to be the goal, because diets are so very ineffective. 'It frustrates me immensely that I see so many women, particularly, in clinic who've been on so many diets – they've been dieting for years and years and years and quite clearly the diets just aren't working for them. They are people who desper-ately need to lose weight because they've got major health problems and yet even with that incentive they can't lose weight. We have to get people away from the crazy dieting mentality and just get a more sustainable approach to it all,' she said.

'The problem is that they don't understand that it [dieting] changes your psychology – you're going to start viewing food as either good food or bad food and as soon as you go on a diet you become obsessed by it and you just think about all the food that you want. And also your body responds by changing your hormonal levels so that you are actually craving more food because your body thinks you are about to starve. It is the natural response of your body to try to stop you dieting.

'Those chemical changes ... Every time they diet they regain what they have lost and a bit more. That's the way the body's designed – to fight dieting. So we need to get people away from that mentality.'

Yet a huge industry has grown up to encourage the idea that we *can* diet our way out of our weight problems. Billions of pounds are at stake and the fashion industry and the media are complicit. So what is the real story behind the success of the diet industry?

6

THE DIETS DON'T WORK

Actress Megan Fox and former Take That singer Gary Barlow are devotees of the Paleo diet, apparently modelled on what we might have dragged back to the cave and cooked or gathered from trees and bushes in prehistoric times – in other words, mostly meat, fish, fruit and nuts. We weren't fat when we lived in caves; that much is true. We wouldn't have eaten avocados either, which are allowed on this regime, but let that pass. Jennifer Aniston, Beyoncé and Phillip Schofield love the 5:2 diet, otherwise known as the Fast Diet, which allows them five days of normal eating interspersed with two of self-denial, when men are permitted no more than 600 calories and women 500. It's a sort of binge starvation, twice a week. Carole and Pippa Middleton, mother and sister of the Duchess of Cambridge, are said to have slimmed down on the Dukan diet prior to the royal wedding. What better incentive than the knowledge that the whole world is going to see the photos?

This is how the celebrity gossip goes and it's hugely influential. Big names shift diet books. Who wouldn't want a body like a diva or a TV actor? But hold on a minute – none of these people has a weight problem to start with. They may, in their own mind, have an image issue, or want to be a tad skinnier for the unforgiving paparazzi camera lens, but that is something else.

None of these diets is the answer for anybody who needs to get their weight down and keep it down permanently. The quest of an actor or singer for the perfect body, with a flat belly and curves in precisely the right places, is a very different thing from the repeated attempts of somebody with a BMI of 40 to lose weight long term and avoid diabetes.

The diet industry, with its gimmicks, motivational books and celebrity endorsements, is one of the biggest frauds of our time. It is not the solution to obesity, but part of the problem. Those who are cashing in on our growing concern about our weight and health get away with their claims because there is a grain of truth in what they say. You really can lose a substantial amount of weight in six weeks. But within six months, most people will have stopped losing it and started putting it back on. It's not their fault. It's the way the body responds to being deprived of food. Yet diets are sold as a life-changing experience.

Some diets are plausible in the short term. If you starve yourself for two days out of seven, you will lose weight for a while unless you compensate too much by binge eating on the other days. Others strain credibility.

I am standing in the kitchen, tapping the left-hand side of my head and neck and chanting. I have to repeat five times (hoping nobody walks in): 'I no longer like the taste of chocolate, I no longer like the taste of chocolate …' This tapping must begin at the temple, and then carry on down the skin behind my ear, down the neck and to the top of my shoulders.

Then the right side. Tap, tap, tap. 'I love being free from craving chocolate, I love being free from craving chocolate …'

This is Kimberly Willis' advice on overcoming cravings (she also advocates yoga and hypnotherapy which may possibly be more effective) in *Diet Coach*, a book that will either sink without trace, like most of the other novelty slimming bibles that arrive in time for the New Year self-flagellation fest, or make her millions. The only effect on me – admittedly a cynic – was to send me rummaging in the cupboard for what was left of a bar of Dairy Milk. This book hit the shops at the same time as *The Overnight Diet* by Dr Caroline Apovian in the US, which claims you can slim while you sleep. One British tabloid got very excited. 'It sounds almost too good to be true but this revolutionary diet devised by a leading US doctor really CAN shift the pounds overnight,' ran the headline on what looked like a news story but turned out to be the blurb for an exclusive extended extract from the book which the paper had bought. Apovian suggests you spend a day drinking smoothies laced with protein powder, after which you will wake up miraculously lighter. Well, you probably will – you haven't exactly eaten much.

This is phantasmagoria. There is no such thing as a quick fix for the seriously overweight. Even the most influential diet guru billionaires, followed by millions, such as Atkins and Dukan, who do talk about serious weight loss to improve health as well as body image, have never been able to claim long-term success for the regimes they promote. Pierre Dukan, a charming Frenchman with a warm and seductively crooked smile, actually acknowledges the general failure of dieting on his website. 'Embarking on a diet by yourself is a huge challenge, as you struggle with obesity, society, your body and yourself. The fight to recover the figure you deserve is too often lost. Eight out of ten people who begin a diet regain the weight they lose within the year,' it says. Whether the 'personalised coaching' he offers to combat this – email exchanges every day full of tips and encouragement at a cost of $29.95 a month – makes any difference is unclear. In a television interview broadcast in 2013, Dukan claimed that of 100 people who buy his books, 25 per cent have maintained the weight they lost after four years.' So that is 7.5 out of 10 who have regained the pounds – not much better than the eight out of ten statistic for all dieters who fail to keep it off which is cited on his website. Perhaps these are all people who didn't subscribe to the emails.

The Dukan diet is high in protein and low in carbohydrates, similar to the Atkins diet, although unlike Atkins, it bans fruit and vegetables in the first phase and restricts fat. Over four phases, gradually all types of foods are re-introduced. Bad breath from cutting out carbohydrates is well known, but the British Dietetic Association, which critiques the most popular diets in the UK for the NHS

Choices website, says it is neither the only nor the most serious issue.

'Rapid weight loss can be motivating but it is unsustainable and unhealthy. The Dukan diet isn't nutritionally balanced, which is acknowledged by the fact that you need a vitamin supplement and a fibre top-up in the form of oat bran. There's a danger this type of diet could increase your risk of long-term health problems if you don't stick to the rules. The diet lacks variety in the initial phases so there's a risk you'll get bored quickly and give up,' it says.

NHS Choices is no kinder to Atkins. 'By limiting fruit and veg it contradicts all the advice on healthy eating that we have tried so hard to pass on to people. The meal choices are limited so there's a risk many people will get bored quickly and drop out or take a "pick and mix" approach,' it says.

But such warnings, tucked away on a remote page of a government website, do little to deter the overweight, hopeful and sometimes desperate. The book launches and promotions, the hyped articles in magazines and newspapers, the celebrity endorsements are all fairy dust and fireworks. When the sparkles die down, there is only the same old hard slog, repeated disappointment and hunger ahead.

If diets worked, there would be no need to keep promoting them. If they worked, the diet industry would go out of business. It is failure that makes the diet gurus money – our failure on their diets to lose weight and keep it off. People who have lost maybe quite a few pounds on a diet, but put it back on again, may blame themselves and return to the diet that once worked for them. Others will switch to the latest excitably hyped fad. So sales of diet books and the products and supplements that go with them are vulnerable to public mood. They depend on public belief – and marketing. At one point, Atkins Nutritionals, the company founded by Robert Atkins to promote his diet and sell his products, was making over $100 million a year. But criticism of the high saturated-fat intake and concerns about its long-term effects, together with the arrival on the scene of alternative low-carb diets, contributed to the waning of its popularity. In 2002, Atkins had a heart attack, which he and his physician insisted in the face of his critics had nothing to do with red meat and cheese. After his death the following year from brain damage sustained in a fall on an icy pavement, the business, without its front man, did less and less well. Atkins Nutritionals went bankrupt in 2005 and is now under new ownership.

The career of Pierre Dukan hit rocky times too. He was struck off the medical register in France – at his own request – in 2013 at the age of 72 after a hearing of the Conseil National de l'Ordre des Médecins. France's regulatory body for doctors heard he had lied about prescribing the banned diabetes drug Mediator in the 1970s to a patient who wanted to lose weight quickly. He had also got into trouble for suggesting that students sitting their baccalauréat exam before leaving secondary school should get extra marks if their weight was within an acceptable range. He said it would help bring down obesity, which used to be less of a problem in France than in the UK, but is steadily rising. In 2012, a third of adults in France were overweight and 15 per cent were obese. Even in cuisine-obsessed France, the healthy Mediterranean diet has been under attack from the modern world. For all the furore when McDonald's first opened in Paris, burgers and chips have become so popular that France became the second most profitable market for the chain after the USA in 2007.

France is divided over the merits of its home-grown diet guru, Pierre Dukan. But the mishaps and his removal from the medical register will not soon make a dent in the Dukan group profits, which had a turnover of €38 million (£33 million) in 2012. The diet industry in the UK is estimated to be worth £2 billion. There are vast amounts of money to be made from the raising and dashing of people's hopes.

When you look at the scientific studies carried out on people trying to lose weight, it's hard not to think that all the blockbuster diet gurus are charlatans – if not, one can only assume they are incredibly hopeful and optimistic people. They must be wonderful at parties.

Because all the research points the same way. It tells us that our bodies, having got fat, will do absolutely everything possible to keep that weight on. It's the fear of starvation. We are like hibernating animals that store up food so they can survive a hard winter. Except that these days, winter never comes. The shops and kiosks are full of food. The restaurants and takeaways are full of food. The pizza delivery is on its way.

The unhappy truth is that when you diet, you are fighting your own body. Jules Hirsch, a doctor at

Rockefeller University in New York, provided evidence in a classic study in 1995 that when we eat less our metabolism actually slows down to stop the weight coming off. This doesn't just mean we run around less as a result and take the lift rather than the stairs because we're tired, although that certainly happens. Hirsch measured the energy expenditure of small groups of obese men and women and some of normal weight, who stayed in the hospital and were fed a liquid diet each day of a precisely calculated and controlled number of calories. When their calories were cut, their bodies just slowed down in every way. We use up energy digesting our food and sleeping and sitting still, as well as playing tennis or football. Hirsch found that even in those passive occupations, where people might be sitting quietly watching the television or reading a magazine, their bodies used up less energy when they were dieting than when they were eating normally.

He and his colleagues, who repeated the experiments a number of times, also found that the mind, as well as the body, was the enemy of weight loss. His patients behaved like people who were starving – they craved food and thought about it constantly. As the Dutch neuroscientist Dick Swaab said, eating gives us feelings of pleasure and satisfaction because it is fundamentally important for the survival of the species. 'We get this tremendous reward from eating and it is very difficult to refuse for some people,' he said.[2]

As a result, when they stopped dieting, Hirsch's patients put the weight back on rapidly, although some people put it on faster than others.

Hirsch and other scientists have since found that some people actually have difficulty gaining weight.[3] Some can eat and eat and gain very little – and the surplus pounds fall off again very quickly when they resume their usual diet. Undoubtedly genes – most likely a combination of genes as yet unidentified – are involved. Clearly not everyone shares this good fortune.

So nature is against some people. They can lose weight if they eat less, obviously they can. But if they want to keep it off, they are going to have to keep working at it not for six weeks, six months or even six years – but for life.

The philosopher Julian Baggini found out for himself how hard this was. Losing 12kg (2 stone) in six months was achievable once he had reasoned out ways of self-control. He loves to eat, he says in his book, *The Virtues of the Table: How to Eat and Think,* but in the quest for a reduced waistline he taught himself to 'urge-surf' and delay gratification. He would note that he felt hungry but not act on it – and in time the feeling would pass, he found. He set himself 'bright lines' that he must not cross and tried to make judgments about the overall impact of eating cake several times a week, rather than allowing himself to be swayed by the temptation of a single slice that, by itself, he knew, would do no harm at all.

And yet 18 months later he was back to his old weight. 'To work, losing weight has to be continuous with keeping it off. This is something Aristotle would have understood. Aristotle argued that knowing rules is not good enough, because we are creatures of habit and cannot always (or even mostly) stop and think about what the right thing to do is when confronted with every single choice,' he wrote in the *Financial Times*.[4] Once you've stopped dieting, invariably you return to your old ways.

People who have never had a weight problem can be cruelly unsympathetic, assuming that once you get used to consuming less food on a daily basis, you won't feel hunger or cravings any more. It's evidently not so. This is how the scientist Dr Jeffrey Friedman, also from Rockefeller University, described the response of the body after a few months of deprivation of its usual intake of food. 'Those who doubt the power of basic drives ... might note that although one can hold one's breath, this conscious act is soon overcome by the compulsion to breathe. The feeling of hunger is intense and, if not as potent as the drive to breathe, is probably no less powerful than the drive to drink when one is thirsty. This is the feeling the obese must resist after they have lost a significant amount of weight,' he wrote in the journal *Science* in 2000.

More recent work has shown that our appetite-regulating hormones can be upset when we go on a diet for some considerable time afterwards. A study from researchers at the University of Melbourne published in the *New England Journal of Medicine* in 2011 showed that hormones like leptin, which tell us when we have enough energy stored for our needs and decrease our hunger, are still not functioning normally one year after the end of a diet.

In 2007, Traci Mann at the University of California in Los Angeles actually looked at the studies carried out on dieters, either by diet companies or academics. Medicare, the federally-funded healthcare programme for the over-65s, was preparing to pay for obesity treatment and needed evidence about what worked. The extensive paper that she and her team published in the journal *American Psychologist* was conclusively subtitled: 'Diets are not the answer.' They looked at studies that had followed dieters over a number of years, not months. What matters in obesity is the long term – not how slim you look for the Christmas party season. They found that a third to two-thirds of dieters regained *more* weight than they lost.

That's a truly dreadful outcome. Most studies of people on diets monitor them for very short periods of time. That's when the results look good. But Mann and colleagues found that the more time that had elapsed after the end of the diet, the more likely dieters were to have put back all the weight and then some. One study was carried out in a hospital setting in 1970, where obese patients were 'starved', to use her word, for 38 days. Two years later, 23 per cent had regained more weight than they lost. But when the researchers came to look at the results for partic-ipants whose progress had been followed up for more than two years, a massive 83 per cent had actually put back on more weight than they originally lost.

That makes diets look not just unhelpful but positively harmful.

And there may be no halt to the rise in weight, Mann wrote. Not many diet studies continue to observe the progress of their volunteers for as long as four or five years, but in those that did, the dieters were continuing to put it on.

Kelly Brownell at the Yale Rudd Center invented the term yo-yo dieting, also known as weight cycling. People embark on very low-calorie diets and all goes well for a number of weeks or months. But then they get the plateau effect. The excess weight stubbornly refuses to shift. Depression and fatigue set in, making it impossible to continue. Weight goes back on and disproportionately what used to be muscle is replaced by fat. It is bad for health and harder to lose next time.

So could diets actually shorten your life? Brownell and colleagues looked at this back in 1991, in a study published in one of the most reputable and important medical journals in the world, the *New England Journal of Medicine*. It's very hard to figure out what is going on with people who are constantly dieting, putting on the pounds and then dieting again over many years. They don't exactly keep accurate records of their ups and downs and anyway, no two people will be doing the same sequence of failed diets.

So Brownell's team looked at the data produced by a large and very well-known long-term trial in the USA called the Framingham Heart Study, which followed the lives and monitored the changing health of over 5,000 people in a town of that name in Massachusetts from 1948. The overall goal was to learn about heart disease, which none of the participants had when they started. But Brownell and colleagues were able to pull out interesting information about yo-yo dieters – or at least, people they assumed were yo-yo dieters because their weight went up and down over the years.

They found that people whose weight fluctuated a lot had a greater risk of heart disease and early death than those whose weight was steady. And this was most marked among the youngest – aged 30 to 44 – who are both the most diet-prone and the least likely to fall ill for other reasons.

While they point out how hard it is to get the evidence to prove that diets shorten lives, they warn of the possibility that yo-yo dieting may actually *cause* chronic disease. That's a devastating outcome for people who may have been trying to shed the pounds in order to avoid ill-health.

By now it's clear we don't need another fad diet – ever. People have been seduced into false hopes long enough. Maybe the celebrities who lend their names and pictures of their barely detectable bulges are dupes of the weight-loss industry themselves. Perhaps they really believe that raspberry ketones will change their life.

Unlike most of us, though, the film star or model who needs a skinny body also has to be toned. It goes without saying that they frequent the gym. If they ever had surplus weight, they have a better chance of keeping it off because they exercise. Being physically active – walking a lot will do – will not help you shift the pounds, but it will help to avoid putting them back on.

An experiment in Colorado has shown this pretty comprehensively. Scientists at the university have been running a National Weight Control Registry since the mid-90s. They have more than 6,000 people on it – all of whom have been successful at losing weight. They all lost at least 13kg (30 lbs) and kept if off for a year before they could be enrolled.

What the researchers wanted to know was how these people did it. They found there were some key things that they had in common. Most ate breakfast every day and watched only limited amounts of TV. But probably the most important factor was the exercise they took. They were all very active, burning an average of 2,800 kcal per week, which is about an hour of moderate intensity exercise every day – more than most guidelines recommend. Walking was most popular. When the researchers gave them pedometers to wear, they found the average number of steps taken per day was about 11,000. These are motivated people who are determined to succeed, but the lesson from Colorado is that clearly we have to get much more physical.

HAES member Angela Meadows from Birmingham University's psychology department believes that diets are actually the root cause of the obesity epidemic – not the excess of junk food around us. It is going on diets that causes people to gain weight, she says.

'I started dieting when I was probably 12, 13 years old, when I wasn't fat. I dieted myself out like most people – if they are dieting they tend to get very big and they get bigger and bigger with every diet and there is more and more self-loathing, more and more blaming, more and more comfort eating, more and more withdrawal so you've got that avoiding, coping behaviour.

'The worse you feel about yourself, the less likely you are to go out and actually do some exercise and people do sit at home and comfort eat and then they get bigger and their problems get worse.'

Her view and that of the HAES movement is that it is possible to be fat and fit – and that if you are active enough, your weight does not matter because it is no longer a health issue.

'Absolutely I'm not saying all fat people are healthy or lead healthy lives but whatever your weight is, if you want to improve your health, healthy behaviour is the way to do it. So for me, I dieted myself up from probably a very sensible size 10 or whatever to the 20 that I am now over the years with enormous amounts of self-loathing – and now that I've stopped doing that it's like I've got my life back. I think of the 25, 30-odd years of my life that I put on hold and I wasted. My mother's 72 and she still won't leave the house unless her arms are covered. She still doesn't eat properly. She dieted all her life as well. She was thin when she got married and got bigger. Generations and generations of women have been wasting their lives on this – and for what?'

Meadows herself was addicted to chocolate, she says. 'I would go out in the middle of the night in the rain in my pyjamas to the garage to get chocolate and eat three bars of it – I was that kind of chocoholic.' It ended when she began 'eating intuitively', she said, which she described as listening to her body's signals. She says she does not now respond to the food environment around her – she is not at the mercy of the advertisers. 'Now that I no longer have that sense of deprivation, I no longer think I should do this and I shouldn't eat that, because then when things are stressful or when that's just in front of you, that's what you turn to. "I've had a hard day, I've been good, I deserve it" – you know – there's this whole way of thinking that makes people very responsive to those environmental cues. If you're actually quite attuned to your body you don't respond in that way, so the environment is a problem for a lot of people, but the environment itself doesn't cause problems, it's because people are sensitised to it for all these other reasons, I think.'

When I asked her if she thought the diet industry, from the 1960s onwards, was responsible for the obesity epidemic, she replied: 'Yes – to a large extent.'

Sian Porter, from the British Dietetic Association, has somehow become the Bad Diet Queen, she told me with a laugh. Every year they put out a list of diets to avoid, focusing on those that have been in the papers and magazines because of some sort of celebrity involvement. In 2013, top of the list was the Breatharian diet – actually more of a cult than a weight-loss programme, but the admission of actress Michelle Pfeiffer that she had been drawn into it early in her career was enough to get the headline writers going. No – said the BDA – you cannot live by gulping air and ingesting sunshine and imagining you are a plant. 'We cannot stress enough that people should NOT even consider following this diet. It doesn't matter what anybody tries to tell us, or point to any kind of evidence, the basic fact is we all need food and liquid in our diet to live. There is nothing good we could ever say about the Breatharian Diet. You can be sure of weight loss if anyone attempted to "exist" on this diet but this would also be accompanied by dehydration, malnutrition and risk of death!' said the BDA.

Even when they embark on a regime that is a little less ludicrous, Porter says people often have a lamentably short-term approach to diets. 'We all have that moment of "Just maybe, just maybe" and "What if?" It's always fascinating that people say I tried the Atkins diet or I tried this diet a couple of times. This whole thing of "going on a diet" suggests it has a start and it has an end, whereas we would say it's about changing your eating habits forever, so day one is the first day of the rest of your life, to use that awful phrase. It is the only way, because if you don't adapt or change your habits then you will end up where you started.'

On NHS Choices, the BDA is a good deal kinder to Weight Watchers and Slimming World, which run similar operations, than it is to Dukan and Atkins. Their regimes allow all types of food to be eaten, but chosen either from a list (Slimming World) or according to a points system (Weight Watchers). Their chief attraction for many people will be the group support they offer. In 2005, the NHS began referring overweight patients to Weight Watchers or Slimming World, paying for them to take a 12-week course. In 2011, Weight Watchers paid for a study to be carried out, looking at the results over 12 months from people who had been referred by doctors in several countries, authored by Dr Susan Jebb, then head of diet and obesity research at the Medical Research Council. The company must have been ecstatic to get it published by the *Lancet*, one of the world's leading medical journals – Jebb's name would have helped. It showed that people who joined Weight Watchers lost twice as much weight as people who were just given advice and diet sheets by their doctor. But 42 per cent who started with Weight Watchers dropped out before the 12 months was up, which is very high. And this still tells us nothing about the long term.

Peer support works for as long as you are peer-supported. When people leave the programme, says NHS Choices, they may have difficulty continuing to eat moderately because they have not been educated about calories. They also no longer have other people urging them on, commiserating when they slip and applauding them when they do well.

The truth about commercial diets is that they are just that – commercial. These are money-making regimes that may do those who sign up to them few favours. The money spent on advertising diet books and products and persuading lifestyle magazines to run features on getting slim buys them an undeserved credibility. Rarely do we hear the truth, that in the long term they don't work. Psychotherapist Susie Orbach, author of *Fat Is a Feminist Issue* and more recently, *On Eating* and *Bodies*, has been saying it for a long time and it's there in the medical journals, but it gets lost in the razzmatazz and glitter of the celebrity-endorsed hype from the industry. And in the perpetual focus on starlets' super-honed bodies, we forget that we do not look like that, never will look like that and – what's more – should be happy not to look like that.

Many of those who spend their lives in front of the cameras do indeed suffer for their art – they starve themselves and experience constant anxiety about their bodies.

Jane Wardle, professor of clinical psychology in the health behaviour research centre at University College London, is unimpressed by most of the diet industry. 'I feel that they are exploitative by intention because they are just trying to make money out of people – and occasionally helpful by mistake,' she said.

She says she feels about the diet industry a little like she feels about supermarkets. 'Their aim is to make money but we've got to engage with them because they are the only way we get food, so things like Weight Watchers and Slimming World, some of the online things – there certainly are people behind them who do have the interests of weight losers at heart.' She thinks psychologists have failed to figure out ways of helping people who need strategies to stop eating when they want to carry on, or not start eating when they'd like to. "We haven't really done a good job on that," she said. Instead, there is just the diet industry with hard-to-follow and confusing advice, telling people to eat this and avoid that.

Ian Campbell, a Nottinghamshire GP and well-known anti-obesity campaigner, says one of the main reasons why people fail to lose weight, in his experience, is that they have underlying psychological and emotional issues that are not dealt with, ranging from boredom in the evening to an experience of child abuse. He told me of a woman who had come to see him in his surgery the previous evening for a health problem, who had then asked him if he could help her lose weight. 'I said I'll try – let's talk about it. How long have you had a weight problem? She says about 10 years. "The thing is, my children were born and then within six months my mother died and then my husband left me" and then her eyes well up and she starts to cry,' he said.

But at that point, he thought to himself, OK – we have something to work with. There were sadnesses in her life that were connected to her eating habits. Tackle those and she may be able to change. Campbell says he increasingly finds that the overweight people he sees are suffering from self-loathing or a lack of self-esteem or mild depression. Some don't feel they are worthy of having their problems taken seriously. The health service is not set up to help them. 'The NHS will provide dietetic services, to provide help to reduce your calorie intake. But it does next to nothing about physical activity and it certainly does not deal adequately with the psycho-social aspects and there's the problem,' he said. He has started a weight-loss programme, which incorporates help for people's emotional and psychological issues from a 'life coach'. It is in its early stages but, he says, they have had exceptionally good results from helping people deal with the real issues in their lives.

Campbell was one of the founders of the National Obesity Forum, but left when it became, in his view, too much about drug treatment for obese patients and too heavily funded by the pharmaceutical industry. There was a time when obesity looked as though it would offer rich pickings for the drug companies. But they have not found a magic bullet for obesity. Nowhere near. There have been plenty of incentives to try, since an effective drug would make them billions. But some of the attempts to find one have caused more harm than good.

Fen-phen is now notorious. It was a combination of an old drug called phentermine, licensed in 1959 for obese patients to take for just a few weeks, and a second drug called fenfluramine, given a similar licence by the US Food and Drug Administration in 1973. Neither drug showed up as problematic on its own or in short-term use. But then somebody hit on the idea of combining the two and Fen-phen was born.

Fen-phen was never submitted to the FDA for a licence as a combination drug, but in 1992, a study was published suggesting that patients who took both pills over an extended period of time would lose a considerable amount of weight. That hit the headlines and doctors began to prescribe both drugs to their patients in combination. This they were allowed to do. It is known as off-label prescribing. Drug company reps often used to suggest to doctors ways in which drugs could be useful beyond their licence.

These days, they are usually more careful. The Fen-phen disaster was just one of the examples of how things can go wrong. In 1997, the Mayo Clinic, a not-for-profit medical practice and research group based in Minnesota, reported that 24 patients had developed heart-valve disease on the combination. Five had surgery to replace their heart valves and their defective valves were seen to have the same, unusual damage. Reports of similar problems flooded in to the FDA, which asked the manufacturer, Wyeth-Ayerst, to withdraw fenfluramine (known by the trade name Pondimin) and also a derivative of it called dexfenfluramine (Redux), which had been used in combination with phentermine as Dexfen-phen.

The combinations had been massively used – between six and seven million people just in the United States took Fen-phen. Wyeth faced hundreds of thousands of legal claims for damage both to heart valves and blood vessels in the lungs and in 2002, agreed a nationwide settlement of $3.75 billion.

The problem was with fenfluramine (and dexfenfluramine), not phentermine. The furore has led to an odd situation. In private slimming clinics in high streets and side streets across the UK, doctors are still prescribing phentermine – and another modest appetite suppressant called diethylpropion – although they are not available on the NHS. The UK manufacturers of these two drugs successfully fought in the European court against an attempt to have them banned, but although they are legitimate, there is no mention of them in the NHS doctors' prescribing bible, the *British National Formulary*. They are given pretty much only to patients in private slimming clinics that are members of the Obesity Management Association, an organisation set up in 2003 by the clinics themselves and the drug manufacturers who wanted to keep these medications available.

Thousands of people are taking three-month courses of these drugs that most GPs in the UK probably do not know exist. Technically they are controlled drugs, because they are chemically related to amphetamines. They are used to dampen down the appetite and kick-start weight loss for those who have tried in vain to diet and take more exercise.

The tale of the appetite suppressants that are used, though not NHS approved, is just one of the bizarre aspects of the weird world of diet drugs. Other pills that drug companies hoped would be blockbusters, earning billions, have also been pulled off the shelves because of their side effects. But patients are so desperate that they seek out both those dangerous drugs and untested, ineffective and supposedly safe herbal remedies online. If they are lucky, the pills that arrive in the post will do nothing to them at all.

Only one drug has official NHS approval – orlistat, sold under the brand name Xenical. But it is unpopular. It works by preventing the absorption of fat in the gut, and often causes diarrhoea. It does nothing to dampen the appetite. NICE (the National Institute for Health and Care Excellence) recommends it for obese patients, but only if they have already managed to lose 2.5 kilos (5½ lbs) over four weeks through dieting. It must be stopped after 12 weeks if they have not shed more than 5 per cent of their bodyweight.

Two others, sibutramine (Reductil) and rimonabant (Acomplia), which were appetite suppressants, were launched with a fanfare and then abruptly taken off the market (although sibutramine remained available in the US) because of side effects. Yet many people still risk their health and buy them – or fake versions of them – on the internet, and some of the pills sold as herbal or traditional medicines also contain these drugs.

Robert Houtman, managing director of the National Slimming and Cosmetics Clinics chain and a founder member of the Obesity Management Association, talked of a climate of hostile public opinion in the wake of the Fen-phen debacle.

'There was a big press campaign against appetite suppressants in the US,' said Houtman. A decade earlier, the death of shipping billionaire heiress Christina Onassis in 1988, reportedly linked to diet drugs, had not helped.

British newspapers became involved and the government, said Houtman, 'decided to get on the bandwagon and have these dangerous, addictive drugs banned'. It asked the Medicines Control Agency to review their effectiveness and safety. But their report of October 1995 found no reason to do so, saying there was 'insufficient evidence of significant harm to the public' from the use of phentermine (on its own) and diethylpropion in slimming clinics. Side effects were 'of no serious consequence' and rare, and there was no evidence of addiction.

Nonetheless, the European Medicines Agency announced it was revoking the licence. Pharmacist Tom Chapman manufactures phentermine and diethylpropion, at his small family business, Essential Nutrition, in Brough, 12 miles from Hull. In January 2003, he fought the EMA's decision in the European Court and won.

'The court case was a bit of a nonsense really,' he said. 'The EU said we're going to stop people making them and I said no you're not.'

Chapman got together the UK and other European manufacturers of the two drugs, they put up £1 million and won their case on the technicality that the EMA could not revoke a licence it had not awarded – the drugs had been registered in the UK, not in Europe – but also because there was no new evidence that they were unsafe. Since 1959, when phentermine was licensed, there had been very few reports of harm.

Chapman supplies the private clinics of the Obesity Management Association, of which he was also a founder member. 'We only supply OMA members,' he said. 'That's been a long struggle as well. Originally doctors were selling it from car boots and all sorts and it was getting a really bad reputation. So we stopped that and said you've got to have premises – proper premises.'

Chapman would like to see the NHS approve the drugs – he talks to NICE and the licensing body, now renamed the Medicines and Healthcare Regulatory Authority (MHRA), about it. But, he says, the private slimming clinics are necessary, because the NHS cannot cope with the number of people needing help because of obesity.

How well the drugs actually work is a matter of debate. The OMA claims a survey of 947 patients at 20 clinics showed they lost an average of 9.6 kilos (21 lbs) or 9 per cent of their bodyweight over 12 weeks – but they get weekly consultations with a doctor and diet plans and exercise as well as drugs. And as usual, long-term data is not available.

Professor Jason Halford, head of psychological sciences at Liverpool University, who has worked on potential obesity drugs, is not impressed with phentermine. The last study on it was in 1973. Phentermine has recently been combined with an anti-convulsant drug called topiramate. The Californian company Vivus got a licence to sell it under the brand name Qsymia in the US in 2012, but it has not been approved in Europe.

There is a problem with obesity drugs that suppress appetite. We know they make people feel less hungry, but we don't know why or how. Halford said scientists need to be sure that a stimulant working on the brain to suppress appetite 'is not doing other things at the same time'. Sibutramine, for instance, increased heart attacks and strokes, although it is still available in the US for people at low risk of those. Halford's group was involved in the trials of rimonabant, which was withdrawn because it made some people feel suicidal. 'We would see people who had lost weight and should be very happy about it, but the drug had affected their enjoyment and other aspects of their life,' he said.

Halford believes drug research is too limited in its focus. Pharmaceutical companies only seek to measure the number of kilos of weight that people have lost. They are not focusing on altering people's motivation to eat or the pleasure they derive from it. A drug would work if it took away some of the pleasure people get from eating or made them less responsive to the look and smell of food – or quickly made them feel full. But such a drug is a very long way off.

If conventional obesity drugs have a poor record, herbal medicines are no better. *Hoodia*, derived from a cactus plant, once looked likely to be the magic bullet of weight loss. It was used by the San hunter-gatherers of southern

Africa, who used to chew it during long expeditions to stave off hunger.

South African government scientists isolated the active ingredient and patented it. Then multinational corporations got interested. The drug company Pfizer collaborated with the UK's Phytopharm, which had bought the rights to develop it from the South African government. Pfizer pulled out in 2002, blaming costs, saying it was too expensive to synthesise the active ingredient, but its lead researcher wrote to the *New York Times* in 2005 saying that they had also found 'indications of unwanted effects on the liver caused by other components, which could not be easily removed from the supplement'.

Unilever, the multinational corporation which owns the Slim Fast diet products, took up the baton, but in turn dropped the partnership with Phytopharm in 2008. A study published in the *American Journal of Clinical Nutrition* showed it did not work – and there were side effects, including nausea and raised blood pressure and heart rate.

But all the publicity, which included TV programmes in which journalists had gone to the desert to try the cactus themselves, had generated huge popular interest. Hundreds of *Hoodia* products, claimed to be based on authentic extracts of the South African plant which is protected under the CITES conservation rules, appeared on the market and were sold as herbal remedies in pharmacies and health shops. They are also widely available on the internet. But most of the products on sale contain no genuine *Hoodia* at all. One study showed 80 per cent were

THE DIETS DON'T WORK

fake. Only very limited use of the plants is allowed by the South African authorities.

Weight-loss pills and supplements abound on the internet. The trade is hugely difficult to police. The Medicines and Healthcare Products Regulatory Agency (MHRA) can shut down websites based in the UK, but can only tackle those abroad in countries where there is a reciprocal agreement. And as fast as one site is closed, several more are launched.

Some of the sites claim to be offering advice and information on the plethora of slimming cures on the web. One such, called Diet Pills Watchdog, appears to critique the different pills and supplements. 'Join the thousands of visitors we have helped avoid diet pills scams,' it proclaims, showing the logos of the MHRA, the Advertising Standards Authority and the Office of Fair Trading. It reviews and rejects a number of rival products, before offering its own 'approved' list, with a link to buy.

The website appears to be aimed at UK customers, but the medicines regulator could do little about its existence if it wanted to, because the site's registered office is in the Seychelles.

'Watchdog Reviews Inc is not a UK-based website and therefore falls outside of the MHRA's remit,' said the MHRA in a statement. 'However two of the products advertised, Forza T5 (which has Synephrine) and Lipo-13 (which has HydoxyCitric Acid – HCA and Forslean), are medicinal and we will investigate these products further.'

In its 'review' of Lipo-13, Diet Pills Watchdog claims the product is 'recognised by The Obesity Society' (TOS), the leading anti-obesity organisation in the United States. TOS was surprised to hear that. It does not accredit drugs, it said, and would attempt to contact the website to tell it so.

Nikhil Dhurandhar, vice president of TOS, pointed out that the website offered a link to a piece of published research on the main ingredient in Lipo-13, hydroxycitric acid. 'I looked up the particular study in PubMed and that study is in animals. Secondly, they have given this compound for four days only. They have shown a decrease in bodyweight but the data is not shown,' he said.

Mike Summers from Diet Pills Watchdog responded to my questions by email, saying that they had taken the TOS accreditation from the website of the company selling Lipo-13, but had now removed it from the Diet Pills Watchdog site. As a result of my questions, they had also removed their 'approved' rating of Forza T5, pending further inquiries. He said the site was partly funded by commissions from products that were approved, but 'there are products in the approved list where we do not receive any payment at all. We feel that makes the site as impartial as possible and gives consumers the opportunity to make informed decisions based on our findings.'

But the positive reviews are written in a heavily promotional way, there is scant analysis of the scientific evidence, which is at best inadequate for all these products, and the site admits in its disclaimer that 'information is based on our personal opinion'. The truth is that none of these products is really much good. They may intend to help people pick their way through the claims and counterclaims for diet pills on the internet – but the best advice they could give people would be to suggest they save their money.

And Dhurandhar at TOS says it is wrong to assume that herbal supplements can't hurt you. 'There is a very popular belief that something natural is harmless. Arsenic is natural. Natural does not necessarily mean it is safe. I would only go by what is evidence-based and one has to be careful about what evidence we are talking about,' he said.

The paucity of approved medicines for weight loss speaks again of the neglect of obesity by those in power. Dhurandhar regrets that there are so few. Even the ones that exist may work better in one person than another – that goes for all medicines. But for high blood pressure, for instance, there are dozens of drugs that work and a doctor can help the patient find the best one or combination for them. Obesity, by comparison, is very poorly served.

'I think one of the reasons could be the overall concept of obesity. Some people think it is your fault – it is your laziness and greediness that causes obesity,' he said. That is wrong, of course, but that attitude, which causes so much pain to those who are overweight, also deters scientists, he thinks.

But now that the American Medical Association has declared that obesity is a disease, Dhurandhar believes there is a glimmer of hope. 'That is where you start. If it is not a disease, why bother developing drugs? All you need to do is keep your mouth shut and push yourself away from the table,' he said.

Drug companies and regulators cannot ignore obesity any more, thanks to the AMA. Nor can doctors, who must now work out how to treat their obese patients, rather than look at them as people with social issues that they are not paid to deal with. And nor can the population as a whole. If obesity is a disease, then stigmatising fat people is even more obviously wrong than it was before. 'Those who did not know should know now that it is a disease,' he said. 'In comedy shows, people make fun of obese people. You will not hear people making fun of those with cancer.'

Of course, nothing will change overnight. Prejudices are entrenched. Drug company budgets are committed to finding treatments for cancer and heart disease (ironically, sometimes the result of obesity, as we have seen). But Dhurandhar's point is well made. It is because obesity is ignored and, whenever the issue is raised, individuals are blamed that so little is done to help. People with a serious and intractable problem which may make them ill and may shorten their life are left to the tender mercies either of dodgy drug sites on the internet or of the commercial diet industry, which sells weight loss as you would sell lipstick or underwear, as something that will make you more attractive and sexy. Oh yes – and it's your fault if you fail, because you can't have followed the instructions on the label.

7

CHILD ABUSE?

In August 2012, a five-year-old girl was taken into care by social services in Newport, south Wales. The child weighed over 65kg (10 stone 5 lb), more than three times the expected weight for a girl of her age. Few outside of her neighbourhood would have known anything about it, had not the *Sunday Times* newspaper submitted a Freedom of Information request, seeking to find out how many children have been hospitalised across the UK because of obesity, with details of their weight and general location.

It made for a shocking story when it ran in December 2013. The little girl was already seriously obese when she was removed from her family home and put in foster care. Her weight carried on rising, to 68kg (10 stone 10 lb) in September 2012, but was said to have dropped to below 50kg (8 stone) a year later – lower, though still desperately high for a six-year-old.

There was much righteous indignation, with commentators asking why the little girl's excessive weight had not been spotted before. In her short life, they reasoned, she must have seen doctors or nurses from time to time and may have gone to nursery school. Why did nobody intervene earlier?

Newport city council rightly refused to discuss the case with anyone, in the interests of the child who must not be identified, but some of the stories mentioned the possibility of a genetic issue. The girl was said to have felt constantly hungry. That is one of the symptoms of Prader-Willi syndrome, a genetic condition that can lead to excessive eating and life-threatening obesity, although it is treatable.

Removing children from their parents because of obesity is a highly sensitive issue and has happened only rarely in any country. Possibly in the Newport case, the parents' failure was not to have sought out the best medical treatment for their child, rather than to have carelessly stuffed her with cakes. But the question of whether children should be removed from their parents to protect them from obesity is increasingly being asked. Some say parents who allow a boy or girl to become so fat that it could endanger their future health are guilty of child abuse.

The Newport child is not the first to be taken away from her parents because she was too fat. In 2013, around five cases received publicity and the same the previous year. A decade earlier, it would have been unheard of.

In 2007, doctors at the annual meeting of the British Medical Association voted down a motion that obese children under the age of 12 should have legal protection and their parents should be charged with neglect. The fact that the debate took place at all showed the issue was being discussed in consulting rooms around the country.[1]

In August 2010, several leading children's specialists, led by Dr Russell Viner of the University College London Institute of Child Health, wrote an article for the *British Medical Journal* suggesting a framework for action – a guide for child health professionals on when to intervene and when to let well alone. Obesity – on its own – is not a reason to embark on child-protection measures, they said. Nor is failure by the parents to get their child's weight down. 'As obesity remains extremely difficult for professionals to treat, it is untenable to criticise parents for failing to treat it successfully if they engage adequately with treatment.'

But there is cause for concern, they said, where parents don't or won't see a problem – where they fail to try to change the child's (and, of course, their own) lifestyle and will not engage with those who try to help, or even actively subvert the process by ignoring medical advice and continuing to ply the child with junk food and sugary drinks. Failing to act in the child's best interests in this way could constitute neglect, they said.

Tam Fry, spokesman for the National Obesity Forum and honorary chairman of the Child Growth Foundation, agrees with them. 'Since 2008 when we started talking about this it is quite clear that something is going really wrong in the family in terms of how the family is organised, how it cooks, how it feeds itself and so on. These children are being fed on junk. What we have said is, as a last resort, once people have tried to get to the family and find out what is going wrong, if they can't make any kind of improvement, then the children should be taken away temporarily whilst the social services go in and sort out the family.'

He envisages the child being taken into hospital as a temporary measure, where he or she can be given good food in proper quantities and monitored. But, he said, parents must not be shut out. 'Parental access should not be denied because it is so important to keep that link between the child and the parent. And in many instances, the parents may even be crying out for help themselves because they haven't got the knowledge, they don't have the cooking skills, they don't know what a potato is, they're really short on income, they may be doing two jobs to just make things tick along. So there's a lot of understanding of this involved. You keep that parental ability to be with the child [but] make sure the parent doesn't take in any choco- lates and fizzy drinks and sweets and things like that. And then when the family home is sorted out, then the child is released back,' he said.

He admits there are problems in his scenario. Hospitals have too many patients already and the child is not suffering from an acute illness that needs medical care. But the intention is to find a way to prevent the child simply being 'yanked away' from the family and never seeing his or her parents again.

This is a hugely difficult area. Most parents want to do their best for their child, but they may not think their child's weight is particularly important. They may not realise their child is becoming obese. Fat often runs in families. Overweight children often have an overweight mum or dad or both and overweight siblings.[2] They may live in communities where most people they know are also overweight. Everybody eats the same food, the pizzas and the chips and the colas, loaded up with saturated fat, salt and sugar. That's become normalised too. In the real world we live in, at what point do you say that a parent has failed to identify and act on the problem and that their child is suffering neglect? And at what point does the child's size, which could cause health problems for him or her in the future but may not yet, outweigh the advantages of staying with a caring mum and dad?

And is it even feasible? With excess weight and obesity now far more common than normal weight in adults, where will all the (non-obese) foster parents be found if children are to be removed in any numbers? Arthur Caplan, a professor of bioethics and medical ethics at the University of Pennsylvania, expressed his doubts in the wake of a case in the United States. An eight-year-old was taken away from his family in Ohio in October 2011 and put in foster care after case workers had attempted to help the parents curb his weight gain for a year with no success. 'A 218-pound [99kg] eight-year-old is a time bomb,' Caplan told an adoption journal. 'But the government cannot raise these children. A third of kids are fat. We aren't going to move them all to foster care. We can't afford it, and I'm not sure there are enough foster parents to do it.'

The little girl in Newport lives just 30 miles away from Georgia Davis, crowned by the tabloid newspapers as

Britain's fattest teen. A report from the Welsh Assembly in 2012 revealed that Wales had the highest childhood overweight and obesity rate in the UK, at 35 per cent of under-16s. It also has many areas of high social deprivation, with families on low incomes or no incomes and dependent on state benefits. Filling food is cheap, fast food is universal and good nutrition was not taught while the current generation of parents was at school. This is a crisis that has stolen up on our children while we were thinking about other things. While children need to be protected if they are in danger, it is no time for a witch hunt of parents.

The Freedom of Information request that revealed the Newport case showed that at least 932 children had been admitted to hospital because of their weight problems over three years from 2009 to 2012. It is not a great number, by comparison with many other medical conditions. It is a shocking number for child obesity. The youngest was a 10-month-old baby treated by Portsmouth Hospitals NHS Trust, while a one-year-old was referred to Mid-Staffordshire NHS Trust. In total there were 101 children under the age of five and 283 who were of primary-school age. An academic paper published in June 2013 by scientists at Imperial College, London, found that the number of young people, aged five to 19, admitted to hospital for treatment related to obesity had quadrupled from 872 in 2000 to nearly 4,000. The conditions doctors were treating included asthma, sleep apnoea and pregnancy complications. Very few – only one in 2000 but 39 by 2009 – had surgery. Bariatric surgery, to reduce the size of the stomach and restrict the amount of food you can eat, is not recommended in children, although it can be considered in those who are mature enough – around 13 years old for girls or 15 for boys – and who are severely morbidly obese (BMI of 50) or morbidly obese (BMI of 40) with a health problem that surgery could improve. Neither surgery nor drugs are recommended for children. Prevention, not treatment, is crucial.

Dr Sonia Saxena, who led the Imperial research, said the numbers were high partly because of better monitoring, including the school weight measurement programme, but warned that their findings showed a 'ticking time bomb'. Weight-related health problems that used to occur only in middle age are now showing up in the late teenage and early adult years. In 2012, there were 500 children in the UK with type 2 diabetes, which used to be unknown in childhood.[3]

Obesity was a word that was once never used in the context of children. Now we hear it all the time. If fewer children in England are obese than in Wales, it is not by much. The Health Survey for England 2011 showed that three in 10 children between the ages of two and 15 were overweight or obese (31 per cent of boys and 28 per cent of girls).

The results from the National Child Measurement Programme, set up in 2005, have shown how early the problem starts and how obesity numbers double between the time children arrive at primary school and when they leave. Children are weighed and measured in primary schools all over England in the reception class and then again in Year 6, before they move on to secondary school.[4] In 2011/12, nearly one in 10 children aged only four or five was obese. More – 13.1 per cent – were overweight. By the time they reached 10 or 11 years old, the number who were obese had doubled to nearly one in five. In addition, 14.7 per cent on top of that were overweight. So nearly a quarter of children arriving at primary school had a weight problem and more than a third had one by the time they left.

Tam Fry says children should be weighed every year, not just at the ages of four and 11. Then it would be obvious that a child was putting on too much weight. 'We do know that the ages of five and six and seven are a danger area, because this is the first time that children are away from their parental observation and they start to get pocket money and they go down to the corner shop with their friends and they pile on the food,' he said. School nurses – if there were enough of them, and there aren't – could pick up on this and talk to parents. Instead, we have the shocking results when they are weighed and measured in Year 6, just when they are about to embark on the sometimes traumatic business of changing schools.

Some of the results of the child measurement programme almost defy belief. The heaviest recorded weight was for a 10-year-old girl in Hounslow, west London, who was 155kg (24 stone 5 lbs). She was 4 feet 10 inches tall, giving her a BMI of 71, which is off the scale. A boy of 11 in Manchester weighed 147kg (23 stone 1 lb). These are extremes, but it is clear there will be many more children who are seriously obese not far behind.

It seems strange that many parents do not realise there is a problem. The EarlyBird study, which monitored the development of 300 children in primary schools in the Plymouth area of Devon from age five to 16, found that only a quarter of parents with an overweight child realised it. Even when he or she was actually obese, only a third of mothers and just over half the dads knew.[5] 'The reasons for poor awareness might include denial, reluctance to admit a weight problem, or de-sensitisation to excess weight because being overweight has become normal,' the study reported. So a child carrying too much weight does not always look obviously fat and may not seem fat amongst her friends. Some parents – around 7 per cent – refuse to allow their child to be weighed.

There are signs that the numbers of overweight children may be levelling off, which is very good news. But it may be only among the higher socio-economic groups. In less affluent communities, the rates are not improving.

Parents get a letter if their child is overweight, which enrages some of them. In many areas, they are offered help. In Oldham, on the outskirts of Manchester, families who get the letter are given the option of a free place on a weight-management course run by MEND, which stands for Mind, Exercise, Nutrition, Do It! The MEND programme was devised by doctors at the Institute of Child Health and Great Ormond Street Hospital. Unusually, it has evidence from randomised controlled trials as to its effectiveness, comparing children on the programme to children waiting to go on the programme. MEND has now gone international: Australia, Canada and the United

States are all running courses, but in the UK, cutbacks in local government funding because of the recession led it to the point of liquidation, from which it was rescued in December 2012 by the social enterprise MyActive.

Just as young children are not responsible for putting on weight, so they cannot lose it alone. MEND involves whole families. Some are incredibly committed. In the brightly lit gym of a leisure centre in Oldham, on a cold and snowy winter's night, I watched a group of mums, dads and their kids running – or trying to run – fast on the spot, breathless and laughing with a tinge of embarrassment. MEND programme co-ordinator, Adele Stanton, had told them to imagine they had just eaten a bowl of high-sugar Frosties breakfast cereal. They were told to run to imitate the effects of a big burst of energy – and then slump to the floor as if they had hit a mid-morning low when the effect of the sugar wore off. Then Stanton led them in an imitation of somebody eating Weetabix (with no added sugar) for breakfast instead. This time the running was slower but steady, likely to last all the way to lunch.

It's not about diets and it's not specifically about losing weight. Children are not expected to lose the pounds. The goal is not to put any more on, so that they slim down as they grow. The MEND programme is about learning to cope with the unhealthy world around us today. It's about salt, fat and sugar, cooking, food labelling, cutting down on TV and screen time and getting more active. It's about re-making your life. Talking to the families taking part, it was clear how difficult it was going to be.

Phil, who was there with his 13-year-old daughter Harriet (the names of children and parents have been changed), was an enthusiast. They had travelled six or seven miles to get to the course. He and his wife were both overweight and he said they had struggled with it in the past. It is harder for adults, he said. The time to do it is when you are young, but parents must set an example. 'You can't encourage your child to change their lifestyle and eating habits if you don't do it yourself. So we are all doing it. We have got a 15-year-old lad who's not very happy with it, but he doesn't have to be here,' he said.

The families have to set and meet weekly targets – eating five portions of fruit and vegetables a day, cutting out or cutting down on 'MEND-unfriendly' food, such as crisps or sweets or coke. 'We are only in Week 3 so there is not much physical difference yet, but it is good that we can get to the next meeting and say I have done this, this and this,' said Phil. 'We will certainly be healthier, even if we haven't lost any weight.'

Nia was there because she thought she was in as much need of help as her overweight son. She had a cabinet with a lock on it at home, containing her cakes and biscuits. It was not so much to stop the children eating them as to keep them for herself. She had post-natal depression after the birth of her third baby and shut herself away indoors, eating. 'It took me 16 months to get out of the house. I just shut down from the outside world. Now he is 19 months old so I am trying to break out of the vicious circle that it was. Slowly, slowly, I am getting out of the house now. I need to go out and meet people and socialise. I have got my confidence back,' she said.

She was looking forward to the session on reading food labels. 'I do the shopping. These are things I'm going to work on – what to buy and what not to buy, what's going to be good for them and what's not going to be good for them.' The weekly takeaway of chicken and chips, burgers and fizzy drinks had already stopped. Her youngest son had been complaining. 'I say if you are not going to do it, you will end up like me,' she said.

Adiba had four children. Her second girl, 10 years old and 7 stone, was overweight, said the letter from school. 'She is the same weight I was when I got married,' said Adiba. 'My sister is chubby and used to be bullied at school and I don't want my daughter to be bullied like that.

'She is hungry all the time. If she is hungry she will go into the fridge and help herself. She will have something fattening like samosas.' Her other three children were slim.

Adiba thought she had herself put on weight since getting a car. 'I don't walk any more,' she said. She liked to curl up on the sofa with tea and biscuits with her children when they came home from school. But one biscuit would not be enough. She would eat the whole packet. 'I have been like that since I was small,' she said. When she was 16 and earning money, she would give her mother her wages but keep £2 to £3 which went on snacks.

Stanton suggested putting away the biscuits and playing a board game on the sofa instead. Food treats set up habits that are hard to shift. Kids buy more junk with their pocket money. 'We have had lots of parents unaware that the children were going out and buying snack food until they saw the wrappers. They were spending money they were supposed to be saving,' she said. Adiba's solution was a money box that could only be accessed with a tin opener. Spending £2 was too easy. When they have £50 saved up, she said, kids will spend it on something more expensive than sweets.

Katarina was a lawyer, originally from Serbia. Her husband Mike was in business. The letter from the school arrived after Stefan, 10, was weighed and measured. 'I knew that he was quite heavy and chubby and we decided to come as a family to improve our lifestyle,' said Katarina, who was small, elegant and trim, although her husband was tall and broad. Stefan, she said, was really dedicated to MEND. 'He has many friends so he was never bullied, but that is what we want to prevent.' In September he was going to move to secondary school, where some children find life harder. And until he filled in the MEND questionnaire, she said, she had no idea how her son felt about himself.

'I was shocked that he would want to be somebody else and to be much slimmer and better-looking. I realised it had been the right time to come,' she said. The children went to the swimming pool for the second hour of activity, except for Harriet, who played badminton with her dad. She said she enjoyed MEND, except that all the other kids were younger than her. In the public areas they had to pass were six vending machines, stuffed with sugar-laden Coca-Cola, Lucozade, Fruit Shoots,

Tango, Mars bars, Snickers, Kit Kats and every other high-calorie piece of confectionery imaginable. Families wanting to change their behaviour need to develop enormous will-power. The world around them is not going to help.

Most of the children they see, said Neil Wise, one of the course leaders, are being bullied. They lack confidence. Children reveal it when they fill in the questionnaire at the start of a MEND 10-week course. 'One mum said to me, "Can I get a copy of this? His dad is always putting him down,"' said Wise, a lean, super-fit, energetic man who used to play American football for a national league.

The objective is to change whole family lifestyles through education about food and cooking and introduction to a wide range of physical activities, including the gym, trampolining, badminton, rock climbing and swimming. On Saturdays groups get together for a walk or hire bikes for a ride. The kids who graduate are encouraged and subsidised to carry on swimming or cycling or using the gym.

There are some changed lives and happier people as a result of it, but it doesn't succeed for everyone and a good number of children regress, sucked back into the world of convenience, computers and tasty saturated fat snacks. 'You can show data that weight-loss programmes for children work. The problem is, does it have a long-term effect? The minute they step out into the street with all the influences that made them overweight in the first place, you're fighting a losing battle,' said Ian Campbell, Nottinghamshire GP and long-term weight-loss campaigner.

Most obesity experts now say that we need to intervene before the age of seven, when MEND and similar programmes begin. Some say that, by the age of five, it is already too late.

'It is very hard to tackle after the age of five,' said Atul Singhal, professor of paediatric nutrition and head of the Childhood Nutrition Research Centre at the Institute of Child Health in London. He cites more data from the EarlyBird study of 300 children aged five to 16 in Devon. 'It showed that 70 per cent to 90 per cent of your excess weight gain is already achieved by the age of five,' he said.

The shocking implication of that statement is that the future for a quarter of children in reception class at school holds a long struggle with weight and probably health issues too. These chubby four- and five-year-olds do not have easily shed babyfat. They have trouble stored up for their adult years. These are the children most likely to become obese adults, beset by heart disease and at risk of diabetes.

In a bid to reach them earlier, Singhal and fellow UCL Institute of Child Health researcher Julie Lanigan launched TrimTots in 2011, which he described as a 'mini-MEND' for pre-schoolers. It works in much the same way, teaching the parents of babies and young children about cooking and how to read food labels but also, he said, 'how to play with their child physically. A lot of parents don't really know how. We give them balls, teach them games.'

Singhal's remark took me aback. In the modern world, parents know how to post on Facebook and microwave a ready meal but have no idea how to play catch. It seemed an extraordinary idea that we could have lost an ability that, if not intuitive, has surely been passed down through the generations. One of the wonderful discoveries about playing with a child is that it takes so little to amuse them. But maybe that was in an era before the instant gratification of cartoons on the TV.

Nobody yet really knows whether these courses for families will do any good in the long term, but obesity experts agree that it is incredibly important to try. TrimTots is one of about 50 pre-school intervention programmes now being introduced around the world, said Singhal. They don't yet know whether there will be any lasting effect.

But this is where experts believe the attention needs to be – not on adults and not even on older children, but on the under-fives. Weighing children at school may give us a better idea of the scale of the problem, but it is not early enough to do anything about it. Professor Philippe Froguel from the School of Public Health at Imperial College London says we should be trying to detect the children who face a high risk of obesity at the time of their birth.

Froguel is a high-flying geneticist, who in Paris in 1992 identified a gene for type 2 diabetes. It did not by itself cause diabetes, but it made it more likely that those people who had it and became obese would get the disease. He pursued his interest in the genetic causes of weight gain and weight loss and found the 'lean gene' in children who are extremely thin. People missing a copy of this gene, he discovered, were likely to be morbidly obese (defined as a BMI of over 40 – or over 35, with related health problems).

But the hunt for all the genes that affect obesity has not yet delivered useful results and Froguel is impatient to help children. He came up with a pragmatic solution – a score-card or check list that could be used by GPs, health visitors or social workers to predict the likelihood of a newborn baby becoming obese. It's a surprisingly simple calcula-tion, involving only the birth weight of the child, the body mass index of the parents, the number of people in the household, the mother's professional status and whether she smoked during pregnancy.

'This test takes very little time, it doesn't require any lab tests and it doesn't cost anything,' said Froguel. 'All the data we use are well-known risk factors for childhood obesity, but this is the first time they have been used together to predict from the time of birth the likelihood of a child becoming obese.'

He and his team at Imperial developed the scorecard using data from the Northern Finland Birth Cohort Study, which was set up in 1985 to follow over 9,000 children from early in their mother's pregnancy. Originally Froguel and colleagues were looking for genetic markers for future obesity, but in the end they found that this collection of basic information about the family was itself a reliable predictor of risk. It worked in the Finnish children and later worked again when similar data was collected in Italy and the United States.

It cannot be easy to announce to new parents that their precious and perfect baby may grow up to be obese. Badly handled, parents could feel angry, accused or undermined.

But the intention, said Froguel, is to help new parents, who do not always know all they need to know about parenting, to bring up their child in the best and healthiest possible way. And the need to do something is urgent, he believes.

'Once a young child becomes obese, it's difficult for them to lose weight. So prevention is the best strategy, and it has to begin as early as possible,' he said.

He was unimpressed by the school measurement programme that may or may not lead to a letter to the parents, advising them that their child at the age of five or 10 is overweight. It's not enough, he said, asking why no central government money has been spent on helping those children. 'I'm a bit irritated to see that everyone talks about obesity and nobody does anything,' he said. 'It is time to try to predict and do something. We know by the age of five or six it is too late. Everything happens between birth and five.'

He wants to see parents taught about the dangers of over-feeding babies and of giving their small children biscuits, sweets, crisps and other junk food. 'I'm a physician and I work in a hospital for children. There are a lot of young women of low income and low education who have absolutely no idea about nutrition and what to do with their child who is crying,' he said, pointing out that the UK has a lot of teenage mums. 'When the child is crying, they give more food. Before the age of two, it is not the child [who is responsible for what they eat]; it is the mother. It is difficult when the child is not happy, but information should help.'

Around 15 to 20 per cent of pregnant women in Britain have a BMI over 30, which makes them officially obese. It puts them and their baby at risk. They will be more likely to have high blood pressure, which can be dangerous, they are at risk of gestational diabetes, which is usually temporary but can lead to type 2 in later life, and they are more likely to have a miscarriage. The chances are higher of a caesarean, forceps or ventouse delivery. But the mother's obesity can affect the baby's development too. MRI scans suggest babies can start putting on weight in the womb. They could be predestined for obesity before they are even born.

Singhal, at the Childhood Nutrition Research Centre, who also sees babies at Great Ormond Street children's hospital in London, says the way that babies are fed in the early months and years of life is critical. And, he said, for years we got it wrong. Doctors, mothers and grandmothers, particularly post-war, thought babies were only healthy if they were fat. There was pressure – and still is – on women to stop breastfeeding and switch to bottled formula milk if their babies do not visibly and rapidly gain weight.

In 2004 in the *Lancet*, Singhal and colleague Alan Lucas published an article that turned established wisdom on its head. 'We said big isn't best and growth is not good,' said Singhal. Babies needed to gain weight slowly. Giving them less food, not more, is the best preparation for a healthy adult life.

It did not go down well. 'We were up against the paediatricians. You can see why. In the 40s and 50s, after the war, there was a period of malnutrition. We had to change a whole mindset,' he said.

The *Lancet* paper said what is now widely accepted among experts, although it will take generations more to change current practice and assumptions, and to convince the public that breastfeeding, which does not lead to fat babies, gives a child the right amount of nutrition, while there is a danger that bottle-feeding will give him or her too much.

Formula milk has a higher protein and energy (calorie) content than mother's milk. But it's also easier for the baby to drink. The baby takes more milk from a bottle, more quickly. Babies have to work harder at the breast. 'If you put human milk into a bottle, you get the same effect,' said Singhal. So the baby takes more milk before he reaches the point of satiety – the same way that we can eat more at a sitting if we fork it in fast before our brain realises we have had enough and we start to feel full. Getting more food into the stomach before that satiety point kicks in could be programming babies' appetites for later life.

However, if we all grew up on an island free of junk-food outlets, eating nothing but fish and fruit and vegetables, this would not matter. Singhal absolutely rejects the argument that this 'programming' of our appetite in the first months of life dooms us to heart disease and diabetes, just as he dismisses the notion that the problem is in our genes. 'There are 32 known genes for obesity, but every single one of them together predicts just 1.5 per cent of your BMI,' he said.

So how much of the obesity epidemic would he say is down to this programming of babies for a higher satiety setting? 'Zero,' he said quickly. 'The obesity epidemic is 100 per cent environmental. Environment is the king here. We are saying that how you are fed in infancy gives you the predisposition. Satiety only makes a difference if you are exposed to energy-dense foods later on.' But if bottle-feeding does interfere with satiety, it is giving us a greater chance of succumbing to the junk-food environment we live in.

Singhal and his colleagues started down this path because of research going back to the 1930s, which appeared to show that if you give animals less to eat – a restricted-calorie diet – they live longer. It was a tantalising thought – that going a bit hungrier might also lengthen human lifespan. In the last century, some scientists went on a permanent low-calorie diet in hopes it might prove to be true.

But so far, there has been disappointment and the latest published research, a study in 2012 in rhesus monkeys, our close relations, seemed to suggest that eating less made no difference to longevity – although it did reduce the older monkeys' likelihood of getting heart disease.[6]

So there is not yet any real evidence to suggest that humans who eat less might live longer. But the work of Singhal and others, comparing the rate of growth of babies who got lots of food with those who got less, has now clearly shown that slow growth in babies protects them against obesity.

It takes time to turn a juggernaut around. It is hard to persuade mothers and doctors that what they thought they knew, based on long-held wisdom together with the deeply felt instinct to feed a child, could possibly be a bad idea. But we are living in a different age, when the food we give our babies and our children is densely packed with calories.

'It needs a huge amount of publicity,' says Singhal. 'I spend my life giving lectures and travelling around the world saying bigger babies are not healthier babies. The Americans are way behind. The paediatricians in America are way behind.'

In the UK, most babies are overfed. The first Diet and Nutrition Survey of Infants and Young Children, carried out by leading scientific organisations and published by the department of health in 2013, collected information on over 4,400 babies aged 4 to 18 months. They asked about breast, bottle and solid feeding and weighed, measured and tested babies to find out if they were getting sufficient food and vitamins and minerals. They were. In fact, they were getting more than enough. Three-quarters of the babies (75 per cent of boys and 76 per cent of girls) were getting more calories than they needed, said the report. In the younger babies, that was mostly from formula milk and in the older ones from solids as well.

And the risks for babies in poorer countries, where formula milk and junk food are increasingly available, are rising. Singhal talks to the World Health Organisation, which has used the team's data as the basis for its growth charts for babies, about the problem in developing countries. Studies in Africa, Brazil, Guatemala, China and India have shown exactly the same thing, he said. 'Faster-growing babies have an increased risk of obesity and cardiovascular disease in later life as their appetite changes and they get more energy-dense foods.'

Trying to protect children from energy-dense junk food as they grow up is very hard. Food and drink companies long ago realised that marketing to children, harnessing their pester power, was highly effective. We have had decades of full-on advertising to children, before the realisation that what they were eating was causing big problems. Even parents who had concerns about what their kids ate ended up buying them treats, snacks and fast food for a quiet life and because the stuff was cheap. And the kids often have an argument that is hard to resist – that their friends are allowed these things. So the junk-food culture grows.

Will the industry stop selling to children? That's hardly likely. It would be a disaster for business. The fast-food chains and snack companies need children not only to pester their parents to buy them burgers and sweets and pop, but also to grow up with fond memories of the junk they used to eat when they were small, so that they stick with their acquired taste for these foods – and become the indulgent parents in turn. There is no way that McDonald's or Burger King or Nestlé or PepsiCo or any of the others can afford to lose the interest of the young.

So the strategy now is to comply with whatever regulations governments put in place, as they have to, but find other ways to engage with our children.

The strict rules in the UK to prevent foods with high salt, fat and sugar content being advertised on TV during children's programmes have been held by industry and by the government to have been a success. Ofcom reported that children's exposure to advertising for crisps, sugary drinks, fried chicken nuggets and the like went down by 37 per cent between 2005 and 2009.

But anyone who has watched a family show like *The X Factor* or *Britain's Got Talent* (viewed by more than 1 million four- to 15-year-olds, according to the Children's Food Campaign) can see that junk foods still get plenty of airtime. As the World Health Organisation has pointed out, the industry is just bypassing the rules by advertising at other times of the day, when children are still watching.[7]

But television is no longer essential for advertisers. There are increasingly other ways to reach children, which may even be more effective and are policed neither by regulatory authorities nor parents. Online advertising overtook TV advertising in the UK in 2009. Children have as much digital gadgetry as their parents and are often better at using it. They are easily targeted through computer games, mobile phones, messaging services and social networks such as Facebook.[8]

The sheer scale of marketing to children is astonishing. We parents mostly have no idea what our sons and daughters are seeing. As usual, the best data is from the States, which has been counting the cost longer than any other country. The Yale Rudd Center reported that six billion fast-food ads appeared on Facebook in 2012 – 19 per cent of all fast-food display advertising. Half of Wendy's and Dunkin' Donuts' online ads were on Facebook. Fast-food restaurants spent $4.6 billion in total on advertising in the US in 2012, which was an 8 per cent increase over 2009.[9] This is what the healthy food lobbyists are up against – McDonald's alone spent 2.7 times as much to advertise its products as all fruit, vegetable, bottled water and milk advertisers combined. There is no reason to suppose the pattern in other countries is wildly different.

Food companies have developed websites that are attractive to children, inviting them to become fans of the brand. The WHO report warned of the growing popularity of 'advergames'. 'Most major food companies have developed game-playing and fantasy video sites for young children,' it said. A site promoting Chewits, for example, had an animated dinosaur hunting out the sweets. The response of Leaf International, owner of Chewits, to such criticism was that other parts of the website contained information on how the sweets should be consumed responsibly. However, the WHO said that if some of the videos or adverts on internet sites had been shown on children's television in countries like Norway, Sweden and the UK, the companies might have been held to have broken the rules.

The WHO was also concerned about links between unhealthy food and drinks and sport. Vending machines in schools were not allowed to contain junk food, but in sports centres and other places children go, they were loaded with sweets and sugary drinks. Food companies were allowed to sponsor events, such as the children's Amateur Swimming Association awards, supported by Kellogg's. Coca-Cola and McDonald's were big sponsors of the Olympic Games in London.

'Millions of children across the region are being subjected to unacceptable marketing practices,' said Zsuzsanna Jakab, regional director of WHO Europe. 'Policy simply must catch up and address the reality of an obese childhood in the 21st century. Children are surrounded by adverts urging them to consume high-fat, high-sugar, high-salt foods, even when they are in places where they should be protected, such as schools and sports facilities.'

The food companies defended themselves vigorously from the WHO's accusations, arguing that they play by the rules and also that they are part of the solution to children's excess weight and lack of exercise. The big corporations have reacted to bad publicity in recent years by developing ranges of 'better for you' products, which are lower in salt, fat and sugar, and championing exercise. No commercial company, after all, is going to ditch its big brands which have huge sales when it is possible to make the argument that they will not hurt in moderation – and that people can choose healthier alternatives if they want to.

Kellogg's responded to the report by saying it was well aware of the impact its business had, which was why it was responsible about its marketing. 'In fact, we think we've got a good story to tell,' said a spokesman at the time. 'So, we have no kid-targeted websites for Coco Pops or Frosties and our Facebook pages are locked to anyone below 16 years old. And our on-pack promotions are for things like free adult tickets to Alton Towers.' Its partnership with the Amateur Swimming Association, he said, involved the corporate brand, Kellogg's, and not individual products such as Coco Pops.

Coca-Cola and McDonald's turn the sponsorship argument on its head. They are encouraging sport by their support for the Olympic Games, they say. Both corporations have a long history of involvement, as providers of food and drink to the masses at the huge events. McDonald's argues that few other restaurants could mount the operation they have run since 1976 at the Olympic Games, feeding millions of spectators. And in answer to criticism of the food it serves, it points to the healthier menu options it now makes available.

Coca-Cola said in response to the WHO report that the company takes its marketing responsibilities very seriously across the globe. It has a worldwide policy of not targeting any marketing messages on TV, radio, internet, mobile phone or product-placement mediums where children under 12 make up more than 35 per cent of the audience, said its spokesman.[10]

Campaigners argue it is not enough and that messages get mixed. Exercise is healthy but you don't need a can of Coke or a Mars bar afterwards from the sports centre vending machine. If you do, according to Coca-Cola's calculations, helpfully posted on their website, it will take you 22 more minutes of aerobics, 23 minutes of moderate cycling or half an hour of walking to burn off the 139 calories in a 330ml can.

Coca-Cola's insistence that it is doing all it can to encourage active lifestyles is part of a growing recognition that obesity is bad for business. Marion Nestle of New York University, author of *Food Politics* and most recently, *Eat, Drink, Vote*, looked up Coca-Cola's filing with the Securities and Exchange Commission. Companies are required by law to disclose the major risks to their profits. The main threat that Coca-Cola cited was obesity. 'It's the number one risk,' she said. 'And the risk is because there is so much opposition now to drinking sodas. The word is out that the first line of defence against obesity is to stop drinking sugary drinks and for the makers of these drinks this is a big risk. There is no question that sales of sodas are down. They've been going down for eight or nine years now. Each year they reach a new low and the companies are in a complete panic about it and are doing everything they can to counter it publicly, privately, overtly, covertly.'

If there has been progress in the fight against childhood obesity, it has been predominantly in the advertising restrictions we now have – although they are not enough – and in the food children eat in school. Jamie Oliver's very high-profile and public TV campaign against Turkey Twizzlers and associated processed fatty junk food made the nation sit up. Even the sight of defiant mothers in Rotherham handing their children burgers through the bars of the school gate, while Oliver called parents 'tossers' for insisting on giving kids crisps and fizzy drinks, helped keep people talking. The sad fact about obesity is that it has not been talked about enough. It is not just an issue for a 10 stone five-year-old – it is a generalised problem of the modern age that needs us to think again about our children's lives.

Better school food, compulsory cooking lessons, bans on junk in vending machines in schools and advertising restrictions have been possible because these are areas that the authorities feel comfortable regulating. The impact is on children whom they can argue it is their duty to help protect. There are other things that could be done too. Why is it so hard to get a free drink of water instead of having to pay, which tempts people to choose pop instead? This was something obesity expert Geof Rayner raised with me. 'We should be getting kids to drink water,' he said. 'That's the desirable thing.' Water quenches thirst just as well as cola. It was good that companies making sugary drinks should sell bottled water as an alternative. 'They don't mind being in competition with themselves as long as they own the market,' he said. But, he added, what's wrong with tap water? Public authorities should be promoting tap water in schools, sports centres and elsewhere.

It would be good to think that the focus on children's health is having an effect. We won't know for many years how big an impact that really is and whether it will reach the least affluent and worst-affected communities. But to get any further, there will need to be much bolder action. The UK is not the only country where child obesity appears to be levelling off somewhat – it is happening in parts of the USA as well. But in some of the worst-hit areas of America, you would not guess it – and the effects of the obesity epidemic on those who have already reached adulthood will be playing out for decades to come.

8

AMERICA'S BIG PROBLEM

People walk differently in Mississippi. They have to. It's more
a twist and a sway than a walk. They have to throw each leg
forward and outward at the same time. It's a slow progress.

I can hardly believe what I am seeing one Saturday in
a hotel in the state capital, Jackson. There are African-
American women – lots of them – heading past reception
to the escalator, who are at least four times a healthy size.
On Sunday morning, they are in vast long white dresses,
with gold crowns on their heads, like super-sized angels.
In the elevator, I ask one of the women what the occasion is. 'We're Masons,' she says with a sweet smile and
starts to sing quietly to herself. Unusually, this is an inte-
grated Masonic chapter. People collect in the huge marbled
lobby of the hotel, which has very large sofas and armchairs
without arms. Men in black, big but not quite so big, are
wearing gold chains of office.

They look splendid. Their size wouldn't matter, if they
were not seriously shortening their lives. Some people would
say that is their business, their risk and nobody else should

interfere. But when almost everybody else around you is the same size, the notion of risk tends to pass people by. Big is normal. And in the United States, more than any other country in the world, the persuasive forces of the food-marketing folk are out to ensure you get that way and stay that way. Fast food, junk food, snack food – they are every-where and the predominant culture is to drive in, pile it up, take it home and eat far too much in front of the TV. In a country of generous portions, where the automobile is king, it is hard to know how anybody keeps their weight down.

Sometimes the food and drink ads are in your face, sometimes they are subtle, caressing and apparently totally unthreatening. On the Delta flight I took to Jackson, there were cheerful pictures of cartoon polar bears on the paper napkins. They appeared on the in-flight TV screens as well. There was mom, dad and baby polar bear – oh yes, and a bottle of Coca-Cola. No, it wasn't Diet Coke. 'Watch our NEW Coca-Cola Polar Bear family at PolarBearsMovie. com,' it said. Save the polar bears, but drink Coke. Not marketing to children? I beg to differ.

Mississippi was the fattest state in America until 2012 when it slipped a notch and gave way to Louisiana.[1] According to a different set of measures in 'America's Health Rankings', a report by the United Health Foundation in 2013, which puts the healthiest top, Mississippi is bottom of the league in 15 of 27 measures, including obesity, phys-ical inactivity and diabetes. The problem is huge.

It makes Richard deShazo feel desperate sometimes. He is a doctor at the University of Mississippi Medical Center in Jackson and one of a group of committed and caring people there who are right on the frontline, trying to save lives and prevent the disaster getting any worse.

'It's become normalised behaviour,' says deShazo. 'When you have 75 per cent of the population that is overweight or obese, the normal person is the overweight or obese person – the thin person is the abnormal person. So the whole appreciation of body image gets flipped.'

In Belzoni, a small town in the Mississippi Delta famed for farm-raised catfish, lives QuaShunda Edwards with her twin girls and her mom and dad. QuaShunda weighs well over 135kg (21 stone) but can't see what's wrong with that because she's not ill. She has high blood pressure, but she doesn't have diabetes – unlike two uncles who were on dialysis, one of whom has now died. She was, however, concerned about the weight of her five-year-old twins. One of them, she worried, was too thin.

In fact, the doctor found the problem was with the other twin, Takira, who is way too heavy for her age. She weighs 42kg (6 stone 10 lb), when the norm for a small girl like her should be nearer 17kg (2 stone 11 lb). Takira has sleep apnoea, a condition common to overweight adults where the rolls of fat in the neck impede breathing from time to time in the night, and she has asthma and acid reflux, causing her to bring up her food. All of these are related to obesity. That combination should not be seen in such a young child.

Mississippi, says deShazo, has some of the lowest health literacy in the United States. He defines that as the inability to make the connection between biology and health. People do not understand what may make them ill. DeShazo, a deeply caring man and a practising Methodist, who says poverty and poor education rooted in historic racism underlies the epidemic in the southern states, is doing everything he can think of to put it right.

America's farming policy is not helping. Fresh fruit and vegetables are conspicuous by their absence. The Delta is some of the most fertile land in America, but it is planted with crops that attract government subsidies and guaranteed markets, like corn and cotton. Switching to fruit and vegetable crops would be uneconomic for the farmers. The corn goes to feed chickens and to ethanol plants, to fuel cars. Bizarrely, in this fertile land you have food deserts.

DeShazo wants to explain to people how their health is endangered and persuade them to change the foods they give their children and the way they live. He hit the airwaves with a radio show and then a four-part documentary on Mississippi Public Broadcasting, called *Southern Remedy: Mississippi's BIG Problem*. On air, he turns into Dr Rick, full of relaxed Southern charm and humour, entertaining and amusing and educating Mississippi folk with not a scintilla of criticism or confrontation. He chats to QuaShunda in her home, admires the old-fashioned family frying pan that he jokes she may hit him over the head with, talks to church leaders who are trying to help but need to get their own weight down too and shows some shocking footage of human fat rolls and surgery on obese people, which he warns in his jolly tones are not for the squeamish. Too right.

He is trying to get to families like QuaShunda's. Mississippi Public Broadcasting has a transmitter that will reach every home in the state, he says, but he knows even the most likeable documentary is more likely to be watched by the better educated than those who dropped out of school. And he is fighting the public perception that fat is just the way people are.

'We are making inroads. It is very, very difficult,' he says. 'If you go to the malls there are these plus-size shops and the marketing of this nice clothing for overweight people has now additionally, normatively, made obesity OK because they're telling everybody, "Look, you can still be morbidly obese – we'll dress you up."'

Happy to go for gimmicks, he teamed up with a pathologist to do an autopsy on a chicken nugget. They bought some from two separate fast-food chains in Jackson, selected one nugget at random from each box, fixed them in formalin and dissected and analysed the contents. One was 56 per cent fat and the other was 58 per cent fat. There was cartilage, skin and other body parts, vibrated free of the skeleton by machines in an industrial process designed to use as much of the carcass as possible. The Jackson nuggets contained less than 20 per cent protein and the rest was carbohydrate. Chicken nugget, said deShazo and colleagues in the paper they wrote for the *American Journal of Medicine*, was a misnomer – not chicken nugget, but chicken little. Doctors should tell their patients of the limited nutritional value of this and other processed foods, they said.

Next he plans an art show. This will be MRI scans of the morbidly obese, showing the rivers of internal fat wrapped round the intestines, which squeeze the kidneys until they are tiny and reduce the blood flow – possibly the reason for the hypertension (high blood pressure) obese people suffer. The scans show bloated livers, swollen by having to process and store too much fat, and hearts and lungs pushed up into the top of the chest cavity. It's no wonder obese people get breathless. 'These are the morbidly obese people we see all the time. We have to have extra-large beds, extra-large scales, extra-large chairs, extra-large MRI machines,' he says. 'The furniture manufacturers in north Mississippi have stopped making standard-sized chairs. They now make oversized chairs and they have to reinforce the bottoms of them.'

I mention the large women I saw in the hotel lobby. 'It's a shame, ain't it? You're seeing the tip of the iceberg,' he says. 'The rest of them are already dead or at home because they can't walk. You're seeing the survivor population.'

Many in the state do not have a doctor – but they have a church. DeShazo has agreed with the United Methodist Church, of which he is a member, that the medical centre will train a community health advocate for every church in the state – and there are over 500. These people go into their own communities and can take blood pressure and blood glucose readings and tell people what obesity is all about and how to tackle it at home. Every medical student is also trained as a health advocate and sent into the public schools to talk to children and teachers.

There may have been an effect already. 'This year is the first year that childhood obesity has plateaued,' he says. 'But there's a problem. It's in whites but not the blacks. The blacks are still going up.'

Outside Hernando, in the north of Mississippi in what is now the suburbs of Memphis, stands the Oak Hill Missionary Baptist Church, whose pastor has been spreading the word about the perils of the food we eat for some years now. The Rev. Michael Minor says his business is not only the soul of his congregation, but also the mind and the body. What started him on the path? 'Sick members,' he said. 'Coming in and pastoring in '96 and seeing members, doing funerals almost every week, starting out from diseases that are totally preventable.'

Minor was a Mississippi boy from a family that worked cotton fields who was spotted at an early age and fast-tracked through the education system to eventually study maths and economics at Harvard. He made a lot of money in the car business and then came back to his home in Coldwater, the next town to Hernando, and the church. Just as he had been before he went to Harvard and had no other option, his congregation was not willing to try other types of food at their meetings and picnics – until he made the church kitchen a 'no-fry zone'. Catfish, chicken or pork – everything goes in the deep-fat fryer in Mississippi – but not in Minor's church kitchen. 'We got rid of the fried chicken and soda. We brought in fruit and salads. I worked on people here.' He had a cake baked with sugar-substitute to see if they could tell it was any different from a normal cake. He got them walking round the church. 'People started to lose weight,' he said. 'Instead of a lot of people who are obese, there are a lot of people who are the right size.'

As pastor of the church, he was in a position to educate and lead and try to make changes in people's lives in a way few others can. 'One of the things underlying this is culture – the type of foods prepared and the idea that if you are not big-boned and plus-sized you are not healthy,' he said. Cooking has been disappearing in the fast-food tsunami. He has been advocating the return of the 'crock pot' for his families – the slow-cooker, where you put in some turkey wings and vegetables and stew on a low heat so that dinner is ready when you get home. He tells them healthy eating is less expensive in the end than junk that fills you up, but only for a short while.

Minor's is a missionary church. His congregation is small, but his influence is wide. He has also taken up the cause of affordable healthcare, winning a federal grant to train people across the state to help the working poor fill in forms and apply for healthcare insurance. He was summoned to the White House to help First Lady Michelle Obama promote her 'Let's Move' anti-obesity campaign, as was Chip Johnson, the Republican mayor of 15,000-strong Hernando. Johnson has been transforming his town, putting in cycle lanes and requiring every new development to include pavements for walking.

When he started, said Johnson, a lean and fit-looking former submariner, 'I didn't know anything about childhood obesity. When I heard the phrase "This is the first generation of children who may not live as long as their parents", it really scared me and tugged at my heartstrings. As an elected official, I feel I have a little more ability to do something about it. I feel like my generation has not done the correct things. We are responsible for these children not growing up properly.'[2]

Hernando is branding itself as a healthy city, which brings young families from Memphis flocking to buy houses with gables and porches and lawns in its pretty streets. They like the walkability of the town, the open spaces and the safety. The mayor has even taken on the food and drink industry, at least in his own back yard. He banned sugar-sweetened drinks and snacks from the vending machines on council property, causing initial outrage among staff. 'I said I'm not telling you what to drink and I should not,' he said. 'But I'm in charge of the taxpayers' dollars and part of that is paying for everybody's health insurance. I should not encourage you to be unhealthy. If you want to bring your own Coca-Cola in, that's up to you.'

Reaching the poorest people is much harder. Hernando has the biggest farmers' market in the state. But although it accepts government food stamps in payment, very few of the people shopping there have them. Johnson regrets the government subsidies that discourage farmers from planting fruit and vegetables. 'We could solve 30 per cent of the obesity problem if we stopped subsidising corn,' he said. 'We're paying tax dollars to subside a crop that is no use. We feed it to animals that should be eating grass, not grains. We put it in our cars. They use it as a sweetener in everything, which is no good.' He has talked to people on the agriculture committee, he says, but it will take a lot to change the policy. 'I think we are going to have to get some people who care,' he said.

He used to advocate a tax on sugar-sweetened beverages, but he has changed his mind on that. Johnson says what he thinks and the people of Hernando seem to respect it. He has just been voted in for a third term. 'Either you can worry every morning about how your actions influence an election or you can stay the course and do everything you think is right and hope people agree with you after four years,' he said.

Cities like Hernando are giving the Robert Wood Johnson Foundation hope. It has been one of the prime movers in the fight against obesity in the US, with a $500-million mission to reverse the epidemic of childhood obesity by 2015 by improving access to affordable healthy foods and opportunities for more physical activity. Dr Jim Marks, president of the health group at the Foundation, says it is the mayors, small businesses, schools and other community organisations that are succeeding in slowing the epidemic down. There are signs of a levelling off in children and even in some places a small decline in obesity. It's exciting, he says. 'We're starting to see this turnaround. It is gradual and it is early and not yet everywhere, but the places that make the changes in their schools and their communities after a few years see the cumulative effects. We also now have a greater sense that we can say to any community: "If you make these changes and stick with them you will see your children get healthier." This is a time of excitement but we have a long way to go to where we need to be for our children.

'It is a lot of effort. It is community commitment. It is the commitment of schools to do what they can, of parks to do what they can, of supermarkets to do what they can, of people who put in sidewalks to do what they can. But they are the kind of commitments that make a community a healthier place to live.'

New York is another country, but it still has just as intractable a problem. As a fast urban metropolis, where more people walk than in most parts of the USA because of a good public transport system, you might think weight-related disease would be less of an issue. But more than half of those living in New York City have a weight problem: 34 per cent are overweight and 22 per cent are obese. Just under half of all elementary schoolchildren are not a healthy weight. Among the youngest, one in five children in kindergarten is obese, rising to one in four among those in the Head Start programme for low-income families. The worst problems are in the least affluent areas like the Bronx, home to a large Puerto Rican community. There are major consequences in diabetes, high blood pressure and medical costs.

Mayor Bloomberg, scourge of the tobacco industry after bringing in an early ban on smoking in public places, has gone on the offensive also against the fast food and soft drinks industries. Some of his initiatives have ended up in the courts – although parents got there first, with a bid to sue McDonald's for making their children fat.

In 2002, eight schoolchildren in New York claimed the restaurant chain had not made it clear that the burgers and fries it was selling them could make them obese and ill. Lawyer Samuel Hirsch claimed the chain had violated consumer fraud laws. 'Young individuals are not in a position to make a choice after the onslaught of advertising and promotions,' he argued. Several of the children had eaten daily at McDonald's for years. One of them, 15-year-old Gregory Rhymes, weighed 180kg (28 stone 5 lbs) and was diabetic.

Although some saw parallels with tobacco litigation, the case was dismissed – but it had national consequences. Outraged politicians who take the view that what you eat is down to you moved to try to prevent any such action being brought again. In 2004, the House of Representatives passed the Personal Responsibility in Food Consumption Act, which quickly became known as the Cheeseburger Bill. It was intended to protect food manufacturers and restaurants from litigation brought by people claiming their poor health was the fault of the food they were persuaded to buy – as long as the food was not somehow contaminated or unsafe. George Bush's White House and much of the food industry supported the bill, but the Senate refused to give the industry this sort of blanket protection. A second attempt to shield fast-food outlets from the wrath of their overweight customers was made in the House of Representatives by the Republican Florida Congressman Ric Keller in 2005. Republicans like Steve Chabot from Ohio reflected the majority opinion. 'If you eat too much, you get fat.

Don't try to blame somebody else,' he said in the debate. Keller, a man of substantial girth himself, wrote in a letter advocating his bill, 'Do I order the triple cheeseburger and ice-cream sundae? Or do I order the grilled chicken salad and Diet Coke? Obviously, my waistline tells you which choice I make more often. But that's the point: it's my decision to make.' The House voted in favour of his bill by 306 votes to 120 but Keller was not there to rejoice because he was having a heart monitor installed. His spokesman, Bryan Malenius, said Mr Keller had cardiac arrhythmia and that his medical condition was 'not cheeseburger-related – but I do see the irony'.

There were Democrats who spoke out against giving fast-food restaurants a get-out-of-jail-free card, arguing that it is safer to allow the courts to rule in individual cases. They worried about the public health signals the bill would send out if it became law. Henry Waxman from California warned that it would let off companies selling dangerous dietary supplements. Bob Filner, also from California, was worried that the House was sending a message that 'the fast-food industry has licence to do whatever they want with their advertising and food choices'. He added: 'We will never control this rising epidemic without greater accountability from the fast-food industry.'

The bill did not pass the Senate again. Similar Cheeseburger Bills have now been passed in more than 20 US states, however. Their supporters prefer to term them 'common-sense consumption laws'. Jennifer Pomeranz, director of legal initiatives at the Yale Rudd Center for Food

Policy and Obesity argues that the laws raise a challenge for public health. 'While some of these lawsuits may be frivolous, others have the potential to influence how the food industry operates. Some scholars have drawn parallels to the role of litigation against the tobacco industry in the 1990s. Although the thought of an individual suing a tobacco company for an illness allegedly related to smoking may not have been initially popular, those lawsuits and subsequent settlements led to the public availability of millions of pages of internal tobacco company documents'[3]

Kelly Brownell, director of the Yale Rudd Center before becoming dean of Duke University's Sanford School of Public Policy, says the notion that obesity is an individual's own fault is at the core of the food industry arguments against government action. 'This libertarian call for freedom was the tobacco industry's first line of defence against regulation. It is frequently sounded today by the food industry and its allies, often in terms of vice and virtue that are deeply rooted in American history and that cast problems like obesity, smoking, heavy drinking, and poverty as personal failures.'[4]

The food-industry script is clear, said Brownell. A *Wall Street Journal* op-ed piece opposing taxes on sugared beverages by Coca-Cola's chief executive officer stated, 'Americans need to be more active and take greater responsibility for their diets.' This position is also exemplified by a debate in the *Economist* on the role governments should play in guiding food and nutrition choices. Government intervention was opposed by the director general of the

Food and Drink Federation in comments evoking totalitarian language: 'Such an argument has a disturbing echo of our recent past and what our parents experienced during post-war rationing, arguably the last time that governments controlled every aspect of our food provision.'

When it comes to children's obesity, however, it is much harder for industry or politicians to make the personal responsibility argument. In the US, as in Europe, that is where the major battles over food marketing have been fought and won. An adult can make a reasoned or reckless choice of what to eat and drink and nobody can interfere. But a child is fed by parents and other adults and as he grows, is highly susceptible to advertising and promotions, to cute cartoon characters and giveaway toys.

Under pressure of public opinion and campaigns, fast-food restaurants have made some changes to their menus and the way they sell to kids. The Yale Rudd Center, which has done its best to shame them into it, put out a progress report called Fast Food Facts in 2013. It did not present a particularly rosy view.

Fast food is hugely significant in the diet of children in the USA (and elsewhere). Every day, said the report, a third of all children in America and 44 per cent of all teenagers eat fast food – a stunning statistic. On the days that they eat fast food, children consume 126 extra calories and teens consume 310 more than usual – so the risk involved in visits to McDonald's and Wendy's is clear.

Some of the nutritional improvements made by the fast-food restaurants have been loudly trumpeted. Between

2010, when the first Fast Food Facts report appeared, and 2013, McDonald's changed the side orders in their Happy Meals so that they would always include apples and half-portions of fries. Most restaurants offered at least one healthy side option and three-quarters increased the availability of healthy drinks, such as milk or water instead of Coke. But, said the report, only 3 per cent of kids' meal combinations met the food industry's own nutritional guidelines.[5] Restaurants continued to offer children large or extra-large soft drinks (between 350 and a massive 850 calories) and large French fries (470–610 calories).

In New York City, health commissioner Tom Farley has been battling hard to make a difference, with efforts focused on whole families, better diets and more physical activity. Yet even here, with imaginative and combative strategies, vigorously supported by Mayor Bloomberg, they see only a small improvement. When I talk to him, he stresses that there is no quick way to do this.

'This is an epidemic that has been growing over the last 35 years. It is an enormous problem,' he said. 'Roughly two thirds of Americans are obese or overweight. In New York City alone we estimate it kills more than 5,000 people per year. We now have 650,000 people with type 2 diabetes, up 200,000 from a decade ago. So an epidemic of that magnitude that has this much momentum behind it is not going to turn around in a year or two. I would say we're disappointed that we haven't been able to reverse the continued rise in obesity in adults, although there's no surprise in that. We do see a glimmer of hope in the declining trends in obesity in young children. The hope is that maybe that's the beginning of the turnaround for this and we will see that turnaround rising through the age groups and getting to the adults. But we clearly have a long way to go.'

If you look at an ethnicity map of New York, however, it is stunning to see how segregated the communities are. The high obesity rates are not in the whites of Manhattan, but in the blacks of Harlem and the Hispanics of the Bronx. One in six adults in the Bronx is obese, a statistic that becomes flesh as you wander along the Fordham Road, a wide highway with stores and stalls both sides, where you can buy every sort of bargain. In the 1840s, it was a cluster of small farms off the Harlem River and home to Edgar Allan Poe. Now it is a noisy, vibrant open-air mall, where passers-by pause to watch, amused, as a dog wearing sunglasses begs with the handle of a bucket between his teeth, or gather with interest to witness a disagreement between three women which sparks suddenly into a blazing, high-volume row.

Fordham is one of the neighbourhoods of the south Bronx where the commissioner's team have encouraged some of the multitude of small grocery-store owners to join his Shop Healthy Initiative, linking them up with fresh food suppliers. Out go some of the biscuits, crisps and sweets from around the cash register and in come fruit and vegetables instead. There are healthy sandwich promotions and water and low-calorie drinks at eye level. Local people in the community are encouraged to adopt a shop, to help the changes happen. This initiative was coupled with advertising campaigns warning New Yorkers of the dangers of huge portions of fries and the introduction of 500 'green carts' round the city selling fresh fruit and vegetables. In addition, the team has brought in 'health bucks' – $2 tokens for the least well-off to spend at the farmers' markets that have been set up.

Yet in spite of all these measures, the decline in children's weight, said Farley, 'was more pronounced in the white children and upper-income children than the lower-income children and that's disappointing to us.' Most of the effort went into low income and minority populations, but it has not yet had much effect.

New York is being made increasingly walkable and bike lanes are being put in, but it is the food and drink that people are consuming that is causing most of the trouble. 'I think aggressive food marketing is central to the whole problem,' said Farley bluntly. 'The food industry spends billions of dollars on food marketing and they use every tool at their disposal – pricing in a way to encourage people to purchase more, placement of ready-to-eat, high-calorie products, often within an arm's length of just about everywhere you go.' And then, of course, there is the advertising. In 2010, the sugary drinks industry spent $948 million on advertising, which was four times as much as on low-calorie drinks and water. Pre-school children see 200 ads a year for sugar-sweetened drinks and teens see double that. More than $4 billion was spent on fast-food advertising in 2009, Farley said in a presentation to a major obesity conference in November 2013.

'That amount of money wouldn't be spent if it didn't work,' he said, back in New York. 'And so there's things that can be done by educating people about those risks, but we do need to seriously look at those marketing techniques because of the price we're all paying as a result.'

Farley's predecessor as health commissioner, Thomas Frieden, together with Kelly Brownell from the Yale Rudd Center, advocated a tax on sweetened drinks, which they said counted for 10 to 15 per cent of the calories children consume in the US.

'For each extra can or glass of sugared beverage consumed per day, the likelihood of a child becoming obese increases by 60 per cent,' said their article in the *New England Journal of Medicine*.[6] It sparked a national storm of debate and lobbying.

In May 2009, a proposal was put forward for a soda tax at the Senate Finance Committee, during a debate on healthcare reforms. President Obama told *Men's Health* magazine that it was an interesting notion. The beverage industry's spending on political lobbying suddenly soared, with reports of an outlay of $24 million from 21 companies opposing the tax in the first nine months of 2009. Some of those dollars paid for the launch of an organisation called Americans Against Food Taxes, which presented itself as a grouping of 'responsible individuals, financially strapped families, small and large businesses', but was underpinned by the financial might of the American Beverage Association – Coca-Cola, PepsiCo and others. 'Once Congress reaches into the grocery basket, where will they stop in taxing food products to pay for whatever spending whim they have?' its website asked.

The fuss died down and the notion of a federal tax disappeared. But some of the concerned states of the union did not let go. Farley and Mayor Bloomberg proposed a soft drinks tax in New York City which would have hiked prices by 20-25 per cent and prevented an estimated 37,000 cases of diabetes over 10 years, saving $2 billion in health-care costs – but the state of New York threw it out.

They also tried to change the rules so that food stamps for the least well-off could not be spent on sugary drinks – more than $300 million in taxpayers' dollars is currently lavished on Coke and the like. The US department of agriculture turned the suggestion down. So they decided to attempt to ban the sales of super-sized cups of sugary drinks. A 450g (16-ounce) cup should be the maximum available. Farley shows an old Coca-Cola advert of a 50s-style housewife, in a full-skirted dress with a bow at the neck and a big smile, filling three glasses from a bottle at dinner. 'Serves 3 over ice – nice! Big 16oz size,' says the caption. And now it's not enough for one.

Farley says the ban on extra-large soft drinks is in keeping with New York's history of protecting its people from disease, which once would have meant ensuring they had clean water and immunisation so babies did not die of infectious diseases like cholera and diphtheria but now specifically extends to chronic diseases as well as injury.

'The rule as passed by the New York City board of health, which is a body that within the charter – city charter, administered in state law – has the authority to take action to protect the health of the residents of New York, including action against chronic diseases,' he told me.

The ban was challenged in the courts and the city lost the initial action. When we spoke, it was being considered by the Court of Appeal. The argument, said Farley, was not whether the ban was right or wrong – it was whether the city health department's board of health had the legal authority to impose it. 'We definitely think it does. The board of health has taken other actions to prevent diseases – everything from prohibiting lead in paint, to requiring that landlords in high-rise buildings put window guards over the windows so children don't fall out and hurt themselves, to requiring the fluoridation of water,' he said. 'So this is in keeping with that history. And of course the board of health also regulates restaurants. It tells restaurants everything from what temperature to keep food at to what sort of material has to be used for their cutting board so to tell them what would be the largest size for their cups for sugary drinks when obesity is killing far more people than other health problems is highly in keeping with that authority. So we're convinced we have the authority but will the ultimate New York state highest court see it? I certainly hope so, because if they don't that would call into question 150 years' history of the boards of health protecting the health of New Yorkers.'

And yes, he certainly agrees that we all as individuals need to take responsibility for our health. 'However, we also think that there needs to be societal responsibility and corporate responsibility during an epidemic that's killing roughly 100,000 Americans per year. We think it's irresponsible for companies to be so aggressive in pushing the products that everyone can see are contributing to that.'

Plenty of other cities and, indeed, nations are watching New York, which has become something of a flag bearer for innovation and challenges to the food and drink industry. Farley gets visitors from overseas. What action you can take will depend on local laws, he said. 'In New York City, we have authority at the city level, authority at the board of health, but there are many things we don't have authority for. So we can't regulate, for example, the products that are sold in grocery stores. We can't regulate advertising to children or to other people, we can't on our own authority tax anything – we have to go to the state. However, we do have authority over some things done in restaurants, which is why the portion cap was put in place. In other places they may have authority over those things at a local level in which case they might apply these principles differently.

'There is another important principle – innovation for new health problems like this usually happens locally first. Federal governments tend to be slow at taking action. So I would strongly encourage other localities to try to apply those principles with whatever authority they have ... We are frequently in consultation with people around the world who are looking at what we do and then trying to apply the principles there, so I'm pleased with the influence we have round the world on this.'

The USA's other important influence has been Michelle Obama, the First Lady. She could have picked any area of good works when her husband took office, but she chose to launch Let's Move, an organisation to fight childhood obesity. When she gave her first big speech on the issue to the Grocery Manufacturers Association in 2010, it looked as though she was going to be St George to the food and drink industry dragon, running her lance right though its profitable hide. It astounded campaigners and critics alike.

'We need you not just to tweak around the edges, but to entirely rethink the products that you're offering, the information that you provide about these products, and how you market those products to our children,' she told the companies. 'That starts with revamping or ramping up your efforts to reformulate your products, particularly those aimed at kids, so that they have less fat, salt, and sugar, and more of the nutrients that our kids need.

'As a mom, I know it is my responsibility – and no one else's – to raise my kids. But what does it mean when so many parents are finding that their best efforts are undermined by an avalanche of advertisements aimed at their kids? And what are these ads teaching kids about food and nutrition? That it's good to have salty, sugary food and snacks every day – breakfast, lunch and dinner?'

But within a year, the focus of Let's Move appeared to have shifted to individual effort, from exercise for children to growing vegetables in the White House gardens. The lobbying efforts of the big food corporations, such as Nestlé, Kellogg and General Mills, ensured that new guidelines on advertising to children drafted by a federal task force (even though voluntary) sank without trace. Reuters news agency did an analysis in 2012 of food and drink industry lobbying efforts and found that 50 food and beverage groups had in total doubled their spending in Washington over the previous three years, from $83 million in the last three years of the Bush administration to $175 million after Barack Obama became president.

While Marion Nestle recalls the 'one amazing speech' that Mrs Obama gave, when she told the Grocery Manufacturers that marketing to children was the elephant in the room, she does not think that pressure from the food and drink industry changed the direction of the First Lady's campaign. 'I don't know whether there ever was a shift,' she said. 'It was very tender right from the beginning and my under-standing – and this is not something that I was involved in at all – my understanding is that the decision was made from the get-go that they had to work with the food industry if they were going to make any significant change. That was the policy right from the beginning and it's gotten them in a lot of trouble, I think. But they felt that was what they had to do.'

The First Lady 'has no power to regulate or no power to do anything as far as that goes, other than leadership and charisma and she's got plenty of both,' said Nestle. Michelle Obama has got people talking and thinking about what needs to change. Until an issue is visible, nothing happens. The First Lady gets massive credit for that. Other countries could do with a charismatic leader like her, as the epidemic that was first identified in the USA spreads around the globe with devastating consequences. The fattest nation is now America's southern neighbour, Mexico.

9

MEXICOKE

Lunchtime in Colonia Napolis, Mexico City. The offices are deserted. It is 3pm and everybody is out eating. Sandwiches at the desk are virtually unknown. The lunchtime food stalls running along one side of the park, shaded by trees, are thronged. Some people stand and eat. All the cheerful, plastic-covered tables are full. There is heat and chatter and the appetite-exciting aromas of fried meat. The cooks are gently sweating in their white aprons and white hats, loading pork and lamb and peppers and chilli into tortillas, sliding more sliced bananas into a deep vat of oil.

Mexicans love their food and are hospitable in the extreme. It would be easy to suppose that the passion for eating, together with the more sedentary life that everybody leads today, have led directly to the very big problem Mexico is now experiencing. It has taken America's crown. Mexico is now the most obese country in the world, according to the United Nations Food and Agricultural Organisation, with 32.8 per cent of its people now obese, compared with 31.8 per cent in the USA.

But it is not the tacos that are most to blame. It is something that first arrived from overseas, not unlike the Spanish Conquistador Hernán Cortés, who overthrew the Aztecs centuries before. It is something that the Mexicans took into their homes and their hearts. We're talking about Coca-Cola.

It is December and the decorations are up. On billboards around the city, a beneficent Santa Claus smiles warmly at a bottle of Coca-Cola. 'I believe in you, too,' he says in the caption.

Coke began using Santa in their Christmas promotion campaigns in Europe and North America in the 1930s. It has even been claimed that Santa was more commonly dressed in green before Coke got hold of him. But the Coca-Colonialisation of Mexico is complete. In rural areas, where there is sometimes still no safe drinking water, Coca-Cola's famed distribution system has ensured there are always bottled drinks. Its first bottling franchise opened in Mexico in the 1920s. Now Coca-Cola has 70 per cent of the soft drinks market and an incredible emotional hold on Mexican family life. No family occasion, no reunion or celebration, is complete without it, I was told by a number of people. One spoke of visits to her partner's family over a couple of decades, where in the early years, his mother always served tea, coffee or water. It became Coca-Cola and, eventually, they would not sit down to a meal unless there was a bottle on the table. Somebody would have to be sent to the store. 'It was the younger members of the family,' she told me. For them, Coca-Cola was a status symbol – a signal that they could afford it and their guest was worth it.

But it's not just about style. It's also about trust. In rural areas with no clean drinking water, bottled drinks are safe. Nobody will get cholera or diarrhoea from them. You now see babies of a few months old given a bottle filled with Coke to quench their thirst. In the fear of bacteria and ignorance of the dangers of sugary drinks, families are unwittingly exposing their children to other sorts of diseases that could wreck their quality of life in years to come and contribute to an early death.

Mexican consumption of sweet drinks is unparalleled. Mexicans drink the equivalent of 163 litres each per year, or nearly half a litre a day. Within that figure are those who drink much less and those who get through the big 2-litre bottles on their own. It's not just Coca-Cola, of course. There are many others, including Boing, a popular fruit drink, and numerous flavoured waters. All of them contain added sugar, sometimes in substantial quantities. Sugar cane is a major crop in Mexico, although trade agreements with the USA have allowed the importation of high fructose corn syrup, which many believe contributes more to obesity than cane. Coca-Cola in Mexico, once made with cane and imported to the USA because of its supposedly superior taste, now contains HFCS.

Back at the lunchtime food stalls in that Mexico City street, I noticed that hardly any plain water was for sale and nobody had coffee or tea. Almost everybody had bottles of sugar-sweetened drinks. But most remarkable was the size of the cooks and their customers. Nobody was thin. Nobody was of even normal weight. In fact, it felt as though I had stepped into a scene from *Gulliver's Travels*, except that here people were neither diminutive nor giant in height. They were just giant in girth.

More than 70 per cent of women are now overweight or obese in Mexico. Fat is now normal. If this were about body image, it wouldn't matter, but it is not. Mexico is struggling with a diabetes epidemic, which affects 14 per cent of the population. In this Latin American country where there is much poverty and healthcare is not freely available to all, a diabetes diagnosis can be a death sentence. It is the main cause of end-stage kidney disease, when the kidneys can no longer filter and clean the blood. At that point, the patient must have regular dialysis. He is hooked up to a machine that cleans the blood for him, ideally for several hours, around three times a week. That costs a considerable amount of money. Without money or the sort of job that comes with health insurance, people die. There are now around 80,000 such deaths a year.

The first warning of what was happening in Mexico came from the Instituto Nacional de Salud Pública (National Institute of Public Health). In 1999, Dr Juan Rivera, now its director, analysed the figures from the national nutritional survey they had carried out. 'It showed that Mexico had really increased obesity in women,' he said in his office in Tlalpan, a suburb of Mexico City. In 1988, only 9.5 per cent of women had been obese. Within a decade, that had jumped to about 25 per cent. 'I showed the information to the former director. He didn't believe it. He said I must have made a mistake.'

Rivera and his colleagues tried to do the analysis in different ways, but the answer always came out the same. Mexico had a very big problem looming. By 2006, when they did the next nutritional survey, there was no doubt. By then, 32.4 per cent of women were obese. The latest figure, for 2012, shows it has now risen to 35.2 per cent. That is just obesity, of course. The same proportion again – 35.4 per cent – are overweight and heading for obesity. The numbers are shocking among children too – one third are now either overweight or obese.

Is this too many tacos? That was not the conclusion from Rivera's nutritional surveys. 'In Mexico, about 23 per cent of total energy comes from sugar-sweetened beverages and junk food,' he said. 'And I think that is an under-report.'

We are not talking about hamburgers, although they do contribute to the obesity problem. No – junk food in Mexico comes in cellophane wrappers in convenience stores. These are high-calorie cakes and pastries and sweets and biscuits. They are processed to the point where no more processing is possible. They contain huge amounts of sugar and fat and they are very popular. There is a cake bar called a Gansito, not unlike the American Twinkie, filled with cream and jelly and covered with chocolate. There are packets of four small cakes called Mantecadas, each bun containing 8g of sugar and 7g of fat. Would anybody eat the whole packet of four? 'Of course,' said my Mexican companion. These cakes are made by Bimbo, the hugely successful Mexican company with a white teddy bear logo that is the world's largest bread manufacture. It sells to the

United States and is acquiring overseas brands, such as Sara Lee in Spain and Portugal.

The store where I was shopping is called Oxxo. They are everywhere – sometimes within sight of another one. There were no fruit or vegetables on sale. The fridge contained numerous types of sweetened drinks, from iced tea and coffee to flavoured water to every sort of (sweetened) juice. I picked up a 500ml bottle of mango-flavoured water from Bonafont. The label says it contained 10g of sugar – but that is in every 200ml. So that bottle, described as water, albeit flavoured, had 25g of sugar in it – more than five teaspoons.

And of course, there was a lot of Coca-Cola on sale. It would be surprising if that were not the case. The Oxxo chain is owned by FEMSA, which is also the majority owner of Coca-Cola FEMSA, the second largest bottler of Coke in the world, distributing beyond Mexico to central and south America.

These stores are everywhere across Latin America, but children do not even have to go down the street to buy a Gansito or a sweetened juice drink. Schools have their own tuck shops, often run by parents or teachers. The soft drinks companies were banned from selling in schools in recent years, but the school store holders get supplies from wholesalers instead. They have to pay rent, which can be as much as one peso per child at the school. They stock what they know will sell.

And then there are the stalls at the school gates, just like the ice-cream van parked in the street outside in the UK. Asalia Martinez Marquez, who had brought her 12-year-old son to the obesity clinic of Dr Salvador Villalpando at Mexico City's Hospital Infantil, said he could not resist them. Brayam and his friends would buy crisps, soft drinks, juices and Maruchan, a sort of pot noodle soup. I asked him what his favourite food was and he answered, with a big grin, 'Cheetos'. He is far from alone – more than 70 per cent of Mexican children buy food at school and only just over a quarter exclusively eat food they have brought with them from home.

Brayam was at the clinic because he had been referred by the hospital's audiology department – his mother had taken him there for an ear problem. He weighed 56 kg (8 stone 11 lb), but had now dropped to 52 kg (8 stone 2 lb) in the month after Dr Villalpando talked to his mother about his diet. She was giving him more fruit and vegetables, she said. But she would prefer it if there were no junk food available for the kids to buy, in or out of school.

On the white wall of the children's hospital department were signs listing the business of the clinic: gastroenterology, obesity and, chillingly, liver transplant. Obesity does affect the liver, causing non-alcoholic fatty liver disease. In extreme cases, this can cause cirrhosis, which might make a transplant the only option. They have not had to do that for an obese child here – yet.

Dr Villalpando, a paediatric gastroenterologist, said he sees about 200 obese children a month in the clinic, but they have to keep the numbers down or they could not cope. Nobody comes direct to him because their child is too fat – most parents believe their child is of normal weight because most of the others look much the same. They have sought medical help for some other problem or symptom of obesity. The most frequent is black spots in the folds of the neck, armpits and groin called Acanthosis nigricans, caused by insulin resistance, which can be a precursor to diabetes.

'We see all ages from two years old to 16. There are some very obese two-year-olds. There is very, very little we can do,' he said to me in his office. I was taken aback by the starkness of his words. Dr Villalpando does not have, in Mexico, all the resources that might be available in the US or Europe. But it is also possible that he is more realistic than some of his counterparts elsewhere. Obesity is very hard to reverse in adults, but it is not easy in children either.

Villalpando and his colleagues have put together the same sort of healthy eating, education and activity programmes that more affluent countries offer, although the groups of families or older children alone meet only once a month. 'They [the programmes] work as long as they will follow them,' he said. 'But then you bring them in for follow-up at six months or one year and almost the whole effect is lost.'

Time and again, in my conversations with those who really know, who are on the frontline, I realised that we are failing people by our unwillingness to say anything or do anything until it is too late. It is so hard to help people who are seriously overweight. It is so important to try to prevent them getting that way in the first place.

Villalpando, like all doctors who deal with obesity, knows that very well. For him, that means tackling the way people feed their children, from the very start of life. He is quite passionate about it. 'I truly believe this is one of our problems – that we are not breastfeeding properly. This is one of the most important public health interventions and most cost-effective.' He sighed over Chile's recent legislation to give women 24 weeks' maternity leave. That would allow them to breastfeed for six months in their own homes. Mexicans have only 12 weeks and generally take four of those before the birth. By six months, only 14 per cent of Mexican babies are breastfed – a dismal record compared to much of Latin America. In the UK, which is not considered to do too well by European standards, at six months old 34 per cent of babies are still breastfed (although only 1 per cent exclusively).

Mexico's children in rural areas have high rates of stunting. They may be overfed but they are malnourished at the same time. Sugary drinks and junk food do not contain the nutrition they need to grow properly. In December 2012, President Peña Nieto pledged a National Crusade Against Hunger to improve the food supply to poor communities and tackle child malnutrition. Increasing breastfeeding rates was one of the goals. But the official launch in April 2013 caused consternation among campaigners on breastfeeding and nutrition. Two multinational companies had undertaken to help the crusade – PepsiCo and formula milk manufacturer Nestlé. Pepsi's Quaker Oats division would develop two products, said its Mexican president Pedro Padierna, according to the Spanish news agency EFE: 'a cracker and an atole [a traditional gruel made from flour dissolved in water or milk], foods that are in fourth and 10th place in the target population's diet'. Nestlé, meanwhile, will offer help to coffee farmers and milk producers, but also train 15,000 women to set up their own business making desserts, called 'Mi Dulce Negocio Nestlé' (my sweet business).

Patti Rundall of Baby Milk Action, which has for years campaigned against the formula milk companies for undermining breastfeeding, was in Mexico at the time of the launch. She passionately rejects any suggestion that multinational food corporations can have a role to play and openly suspects their motives. She ended up denouncing the two companies' involvement on TV and the front pages of newspapers. It was 'shocking and sad' that the president had allowed his important crusade against hunger to be captured by big food corporations like Nestlé, she said. Their involvement would undermine confidence in fresh fruit and vegetables and breastfeeding, she claimed.[1]

So what should be done to protect children? In Mexico, with its devotion to soft drinks, there seemed one obvious route to try: a soda tax.

In 2008, the National Institute of Public Health published a paper in the *Journal of Nutrition* demonstrating that the demand for sweetened soft drinks was elastic. If the price were increased, people would buy fewer of them. Juan Rivera and colleagues felt this was the way for Mexico to go. And no – he rejected any accusation that this was unjustifiable interference in the free market and people's lives. There is a quote he uses as a riposte to such suggestions. 'Sugar, rum and tobacco are commodities which are nowhere necessaries of life, which are become objects of almost universal consumption and which are, therefore, extremely proper subjects of taxation.' That was Adam Smith in *The Wealth of Nations* in 1776.

The idea was briefly floated by the Calderón government of 2006 to 2012 and got nowhere. But it was taken up in a big way by the nascent consumer movement. Alejandro Calvillo, co-founder of Greenpeace in Mexico, left it after 12 years in 2006 to start a new organisation called El Poder del Consumidor (Consumer Power). Alarmed by the 40 per cent rise in obesity in children since 1999, he started campaigning on issues such as marketing to children, food in schools, labelling and a soda tax. From the beginning, they proposed that the money raised should be used to provide drinking water in schools. Some schools had no drinking water at all. Some whole communities had no drinking water and it had to be trucked in. Deliveries of Coca-Cola were more reliable. Calvillo worked with other NGOs and academics and an umbrella group, the Nutritional Health Alliance, was formed. They sought a politician to champion a bill in Congress.

Marcela Torres Peimbert, the slim and elegant senator who represents the north-central state of Querétaro, was late for our meeting because she had been battling with opposing parties over the poor representation of women in the Mexican Congress. She raced into the room holding out her hands in a gesture of prayer, saying 'Sorry, sorry, sorry' with an apologetic smile. She is engaging, dynamic and tough. This was the politician that the Alliance approached. They chose well. Torres Peimbert was not afraid of a fight either with opposing politicians or her own party. She got both.

When I asked why she proposed the tax, she reeled off the figures – the deaths, the soaring costs of obesity-associated healthcare, predicted to rise from 80 billion pesos a year in 2012 to 150 billion in 2017. 'I agreed to present it first because it will save lives,' she said. 'Both my parents and my sisters are doctors. I have been very conscious of weight and diabetes and the obesity problem.' While she was a member of her state government, she had charge of the social programmes, which included a rehabilitation centre where 70 per cent of the patients were suffering from the consequences of diabetes or stroke as a result of high blood pressure caused by obesity.

Torres Peimbert talks of Coca-Cola's dominance in the country, of the Oxxo stores which sell only processed food, of the company sponsorship of football pitches and how it paid for the infrastructure of little stores in schools, all carrying the company logo, where children would buy junk food and sweet drinks. 'We have to regulate the food sold in schools,' she said. There is a voluntary agreement that they will sell healthy products, but the need to make a profit undermines that. 'The stores in the schools are owned by the teachers, but they don't have water and they just sell junk food. We took that away in 60 schools in my state and the children started seeing low-sugar, low-fat produce. Those were the only things children in those schools could buy. The children responded. They had mango, yoghurt and plain and fruit water. They bought these things and we also had less sickness in the stomach because we forced them [the teachers running the stores] to have running water [to wash their hands].'

Torres Peimbert is a member of PAN (the National Action Party), which is not in the majority, nor the party of the president. It is the party of a former president, Vicente Fox, who ran the country from 2000 to 2006, and who was the first in 71 years to defeat the candidate of the dominant Institutional Revolutionary Party (PRI). But ironically, before he went into politics, Fox was president of a different sort – he ran Coca-Cola Mexico, where he increased sales by 50 per cent and expanded its hold on other countries in Latin America. 'We owed democracy in part to Coca-Cola,' Torres Peimbert exclaimed. 'He is a wonderful person, but he was their national director.' Fox, who started out driving trucks for Coke in 1964, climbed up the company ladder and made the sort of fortune that allowed him to stand for the highest office in the land.

When Torres Peimbert agreed to present a bill to Congress to impose a tax on sweetened soft drinks, she knew she would have to confront all kinds of vested interests. 'I knew the consequences would be unpopular,' she said. 'The industry spends a lot of time and money on politics in Mexico. They pay for campaigns of every political party.

They give private donations. They don't have a particular ideology.' It is all open and legitimate. Some parliamentarians also have business interests themselves in soft drinks, a fact which is known and does not debar them from taking the industry's side.

Industry lobbyists came to see Torres Peimbert, naturally. They came armed with studies the companies had themselves funded to try to prove sugar-sweetened drinks did no harm. They argued that jobs would be lost in the soft drinks factories, the sugar cane plantations and shops. But, she said, by then she had 'a deep knowledge of the problem', and they left unsatisfied.

'I wasn't threatened, but in a way I was, because I received two calls from regional owners where I live. They said we have been your friends. I have never received a peso from them, but they have helped my political party and other colleagues. I told them I'm not trying to do you any harm – just trying to improve the health of my country.'

Her own party would not support her, 'because it will be read as PAN against the soda industry'. She was blocked and discussion of her bill was delayed, time and again, by her colleagues. Eventually she managed to present it and was told by her party that it would not be passed. The bill ultimately fell, but it succeeded in raising considerable debate about the tax in and outside of Congress.

Meanwhile, out on the traffic-thronged streets of Mexico City, a battle of the billboards had broken out. The Nutritional Health Alliance launched a groundbreaking advertising campaign on a scale and level of sophistication that had not been seen before in support of a health or social cause.

The first the people of Mexico knew of it, as they sat stuck in traffic in the autumn of 2012, was the shocking picture of a man sitting in a wheelchair with parts of his feet missing as a result of diabetes. 'First came obesity. Then diabetes. What was the contribution of soft drinks advertising?' ran the slogan. Two more ads ran on the same theme – one showing somebody who has gone blind as a result of the disease and the other showing the foot of a corpse, with a tag tied to the toe saying 'diabetes'.

But it was a subtler advert that caused the biggest stir. Between May and August 2013, posters went up showing the trusting faces of two children, looking up at an unseen adult handing them a bottle. 'Would you give them 12 spoonfuls of sugar?' the caption asked. 'Why do you give them soft drinks?' People had been unaware of the quantity of sugar in a 600ml bottle of sweetened drink. The campaigners linked sugary drinks to disease. 'Soda is sweet – diabetes isn't,' said the ads. The concept of unwittingly harming one's own children struck a chord.

The Alliance was able to run this sort of campaign only because it had a substantial war chest in the shape of financial support from US-based Bloomberg Philanthropies, which had already been working on its principal concern, tobacco control, with some of the same NGOs in Mexico, and also ran campaigns outside the United States on road safety. The foundation decided it made sense to extend its activities to the prevention of obesity, a growing menace to world health. Mexico was a neighbour, and the NGOs were known and trusted. After many months of discussions, the decision was made to finance their efforts, focusing on the soda tax campaign, the marketing of junk food to children and better nutrition labelling.

But there was clearly a risk. Nobody can deny the deadly nature of tobacco. There is nothing good to be said about cigarettes. But we need food and drink. Experts hired by industry argue – and governments like that in the UK buy the argument – that there is nutritional value in anything, as long as you don't have too much of it. If you need 2,000 calories a day, theoretically you can get them from any source. So who are Bloomberg Philanthropies, the Mexican soft drinks industry was quick to ask, to tell us what to consume? In their own advertising campaign, countering that of the Alliance, they dubbed the proposed levy 'the Bloomberg tax' and linked it to the Mayor of New York who had failed to ban super-sized cups of soda in his own city, rather than to the charitable foundation he supports. 'NO TO THE BLOOMBERG TAX,' shouted the billboards. 'Michael Bloomberg, Mayor of New York, has financed with $10 million a health campaign against sugary drinks. He wants to do in Mexico what he could not do in the United States.' An anonymous video appeared on the internet featuring pictures of Alejandro Calvillo with Michael Bloomberg. It asked, 'Do you want gringos telling you what to do?'

The claim that a foreigner was interfering in Mexico because he could not get his own way in his own country ran in the papers for a couple of weeks. 'I think it's not unexpected,' said Dr Kelly Henning, who runs public health programmes at Bloomberg Philanthropies. 'I think the partners anticipated that was one of the tactics the food and beverage industry would use to push back against the taxes. They were very much trying to grab onto any possible counter-argument that they could pose and that was one that was expected somewhat. I think the partners did a really great job of getting their message out – which was how harmful sugar-sweetened beverages have become for the Mexican population and what phenomenally large amounts are being consumed.'

When I met Jorge Romo, the corporate lawyer who speaks for the Asociación Nacional de Productores de Refrescos y Aguas Carbonatadas (ANPRAC) – the soft drinks manufacturers – he raised the issue before I could. 'And now let's talk about Mr Bloomberg,' he said. 'He is investing $10m for this campaign, against mainly Coca-Cola. Maybe he has a reason. We say that he failed in New York to put in that programme limiting sizes, so why come to Mexico to bring his programme?

'We saw the difference between before maybe last year, and now. Their advertisements are all over – in school these sorts of huge announcements, huge signs, on the radio, in some TV channels, mainly directly on the streets – don't consume sugary drinks, they are harmful for your health.'

But aren't they harmful to your health, I asked Romo? 'I'm not in the medical area, so I cannot affirm or deny that problem, but we think in accordance with our experts in this area that that is not the main cause of the problem in

Mexico,' he said. 'The main cause is that we have a Latin gene that produces the problem mainly. Secondly, the type of food that Mexicans eat – saturated fat all over in every corner. You can see just here, around the corner – these stands in the street. This is unnecessary industrialised food, packaged food.'

Romo also blamed poverty – although Juan Rivera at the National Institute of Health has shown that Mexico does not have the same pattern as the wealthiest countries, where the rich are thinnest and the poor suffer most from obesity. Rivera's figures show obesity is remarkably consistent in Mexico, from rich to poor and from rural village to city centre.

But it was not Romo's argument. 'The problem mainly is poverty,' said the corporate lawyer, who is a substantial figure himself, sitting in the upmarket hotel restaurant where I had invited him for coffee. Toying with a bun, he said, 'They cannot afford better food. They cannot go to their homes to have food at dinner time or lunch time so it is a big problem. They don't eat fruit, they don't eat vegetables. So they only eat carbohydrates.'

A soda tax, in his view, would penalise these same people. The poorest spend 6 per cent of their income on soft drinks, he said – a significant slice. But that's the point, I said. If these drinks become more expensive, people will buy fewer of them. They are not an essential, like water. It worked with cigarettes – the higher the price goes, the more people try to cut down. It should be easier with soft drinks. Even if sugar is a bit addictive, it's not like nicotine.

Romo was having none of it. The tax won't work, in his view. It may have an impact for the first few months, but in the long term it will not reduce consumption by more than 1 per cent at best, he claimed. The increased cost of soft drinks will just be a further burden on the poor. He did not deny obesity is a problem, but it needs to be tackled by targeting junk food and promoting exercise, instead of picking on the most visible target – the soft drinks companies, with Coca-Cola at their head, sporting the most famous red logo in the world.

The Alliance's billboard and subway adverts did very well. Polling showed that 59 per cent of people who saw the 12 spoonfuls of sugar poster said they tried to give their children fewer soft drinks afterwards and 44 per cent said they themselves drank less as a result. But when the NGOs tried to take the message to television, to reach substantially more of Mexico's 118 million population, they hit a wall.

There had been a hint of what might happen. One of the billboard companies had refused to run some campaign ads and they were also turned away by a publicity organisation for the main public bus stop sites. But that was little more than an inconvenience – there were other outlets. Being blocked by the TV companies, as they found they were, was far more problematic. Two companies, Televisa and TV Azteca, between them control about 90 per cent of national public broadcasting. On 21 August 2013, ahead of Congress voting on the soda tax, the Alliance requested airtime for its adverts. The TV companies refused. They would not meet to discuss their reasons and they would put nothing in writing.

On 8 September, President Enrique Peña Nieto, who had pledged support for a soda tax before his election, officially presented to Congress a package of fiscal reform which included the tax. With this backing from the head of state, it looked as though one of the TV stations was going to back down. 'We received a call from TV Azteca informing us that they would be happy to run the ad,' said Rebecca Berner from El Poder del Consumidor. 'In a formal meeting with their executives on 18 September, although insisting that [the Alliance] had to pay a full rate [at government prices, the highest on their scale], we made a verbal agreement to run the ad. On 25 September, after follow-up dialogues and discussions on the details of schedules, TV Azteca informed us with a phone call that they had no available airtime on any station through December for our ad.'

'Given this blockage by the main TV companies, on 2 September, we contacted Milenio TV, the company with the third most important nightly news programme. All preparations were underway, including the delivery of the commercial, but on the evening of 3 September, we were informed they had no available airtime at any time for our commercial.'

They went to cable TV instead and encountered no obstacles. The Alliance is outraged that they were blocked by the mainstream companies. On 30 September, they ran adverts denouncing them, under a picture of a small girl drinking from a water fountain. 'What is more important:

public health or the interests of the soft drinks companies?' it asked, above a link to a web page. 'Watch the advert that Televisa, TV Azteca and Milenio TV refused to show.'

Emails to all three companies received no response. When I mentioned the TV companies' refusal to air the soda tax campaign ads to Romo, he shrugged. Maybe they had advertising contracts with the soft drinks companies, he said.

Despite the corporate opposition, the tax was passed by Congress on 31 October, at the rate of one peso on every litre of sugar-sweetened drink, or roughly 10 per cent. That means it will affect flavoured waters equally as much as Coca-Cola and Boing. A tax on junk food was also passed, at 8 per cent for products containing 275 calories or more per 100g. On the same day, President Peña Nieto announced a national strategy to prevent and treat obesity and diabetes. To the surprise of all of the campaigners, when Peña Nieto sat down, Brian Smith, president of the Coca-Cola Company Group in Latin America stood up. He pledged to focus on sales of low-calorie and no-calorie drinks, improve the transparency of labelling and not market to children under 12.

These are familiar lines in Europe and the USA, where labelling is a big issue and the move to low-calorie drinks is growing, but there is considerable work to do in Mexico. Juan Rivera has a slide he shows of a Coca-Cola advert which appeared in the *Reforma* newspaper in August 2010 to illustrate unethical marketing. It shows the dietary information on a familiar red can of Coca-Cola as sold by the Mexican corporation. Under the slogan, 'Nothing to hide', the ad states that 200ml of Coke, containing 21g of sugar, provides only 17 per cent of the recommended daily sugar intake. But that's according to Coca-Cola Mexico's own preferred daily limit of 25 per cent of energy from sugar per day. The World Health Organisation's guideline says no more than 10 per cent.

And that assumes you drink not much more than half the can. The whole can contains 37g of sugar. By WHO standards that's three-quarters of your day's sugar in one can. 'So, nothing to hide, really?' asks Rivera.

Many anti-obesity campaigners believe the tax could and should have been higher. Alejandro Calvillo and the rest of the Alliance wanted a tax of 20 per cent, which they believe would have made a real impact. Rivera and colleagues at the National Institute of Public Health estimate it would cut sugared drinks consumption from 163 litres per person per year to somewhere between 121 and 130 litres per person, and raise 22 to 24 billion pesos – over £1 billion. A 10 per cent tax would bring consumption down to between 141 and 146 litres per person, they estimate, and raise 15 to 16 billion pesos – between £700 and £750 million.

For Marcela Torres Peimbert, one of the most critical issues now is ensuring that the money raised is spent in those schools that have no clean water for children to drink. 'The tax passed, but I don't trust my government to use the money from the tax for health in Mexico,' she said. 'It has to be spent on three things – water for the public schools, water for poor communities and education for the prevention of obesity, overweight and diabetes.' For the credibility of the tax, the money needs to be used in the way that was promised. Polling showed that people approved of the price increase in soda as long as it was to be spent on water fountains and filtration systems. But taxes in Mexico have not previously been earmarked for specific purposes and there are concerns that a cash-strapped government may prefer to add the money to its general spending pool, if it can get away with it.

In general, though, the civil society organisations which did battle on the advertising hoardings and through demonstrations, street events and press conferences were just delighted that the tax was passed. 'It is very, very important not only for Mexico,' said Calvillo, director of El Poder del Consumidor. 'It is an issue that has an international resonance. I was very happy [when it was passed] but at the same time I felt a growing sense of responsibility because we know the reality of this country. We know that there are people who drink a lot of sodas and they don't have access to drinking water. A very great concern was to gain support for this tax for drinking water inside schools so that part of the resources from the soda tax and tax on junk food go to health issues.'

And he does not believe the fight with the drinks industry is over yet. There is too much at stake. 'In reality when you talk about sweetened beverages in Mexico, you talk about Coke. They have 70 per cent. They will do anything to kill this tax.'

It matters even more because the Mexico tax is a precedent for the whole world. So far, the soft drinks industry globally has been able to say there is no proof it will reduce obesity and diseases like diabetes. If Mexico proves them wrong, other countries will have an incentive to raise taxes on sugary drinks too. Tom Farley, health commissioner of New York City, said many in the USA were watching closely. 'I am hopeful though that with the passage of that in Mexico, when people see the benefits of that, legislatures around the country will be supportive of it. I can't say whether we're going to be the first place to do it in the US. There are many places looking at it. … I'm hopeful that some places in the US will now work harder at achieving it and when they do, other places will be having a new go at passing it.'

Bloomberg Philanthropies will also be paying close attention. 'When the numbers are so large we're imagining we will be able to see impact,' said Henning. 'The larger the tax, the greater the impact, but I think people are very hopeful this will be sufficient to demonstrate real change.'

For them, the Mexican programme they funded is a pilot. If all goes well, they will consider helping civil society organisations in other countries to mount similar campaigns, although Henning is cautious. 'We haven't formed a Plan B yet – a next phase. I can say that in the road safety programme, for example, we did a two-year pilot in Vietnam and Mexico which we felt was very successful and we built it on that to develop a ten-country, five-year multimillion dollar programme. We're hoping that this will be successful and it will lead us to more opportunity in this area. I can't say for sure whether that's going to be the case but it's sort of the way in which we work.'

There could be plenty of openings for Bloomberg if it wants them. There is real concern in many middle-income countries. Enrique Jacoby, regional advisor on healthy eating and active living to the Pan American Health Organisation, says Mexico's high obesity rates have attracted a lot of attention, but it is a similar story all over Latin America. Traditional diets have been ousted by 'ultra-processed' food. Surveys of people's shopping habits show that in Chile, too, close to half of all the food bought to eat in the home is junk food, Jacoby said. It has displaced the whole grains, lentils, fruit, vegetables and meat that people used to cook.

But, said Jacoby, there is a resistance movement. It is called mothers and grandmothers. 'They still know what is good food and what is junk. They fight back so their kids don't consume junk all the time.' It is a battle that needs to be fought. He compared what has happened in the United States. 'The US has lost the ability to prepare whole food for three generations in a row. People are being fed by industry. This progression is terrible. In Latin America, we have amazing culinary traditions which provide for our nourishment. There is a lot of praise for it internationally, but we are losing it as we speak,' he said. And children's appreciation of the taste of good food never properly develops.

There is growing public awareness of the peril that Latin America is in and countries have been trying to regulate as a result – sometimes taking a tougher stand than Europe or the USA has managed. Mexico's soda tax is an example and so is the law that Ecuador passed at the end of 2013, bringing in the world's first mandatory traffic light food labelling. The UK version, on which it is modelled, is only voluntary. Latin America seems less impressed with industry self-regulation and voluntary approaches.

Chile brought in a labelling and marketing law, which among other things banned toys, crayons and stickers from boxes of cereal and fast food – a measure the companies thwarted in the USA by making a small charge for them. Peru passed extensive regulations to curb the advertising of foods and drinks high in trans fat, saturated fat, sugar and salt. Adverts are not permitted that suggest a parent is more intelligent or more generous if he or she buys a certain product, or that appeal to a child's emotions. Adverts were also banned that encouraged children to eat large portions of processed food or sweet drinks. School kiosks were ordered to dump the junk and sell only healthy food instead.

But passing a law is one thing and getting it implemented has turned out to be another. The food and drink companies, according to Jacoby, have been very adept at delaying implementation, so that the new rules sit on the statute books and no more. They spend a fortune on lobbyists and lawyers and throw at ministers the same arguments heard in Mexico – that people will lose jobs if the food and drink industries lose sales.

In Brazil, the industry line is generally supported by the press, he says, which means that criticism does not get heard. So Carlos Monteiro from the University of São Paulo, one of the biggest critics of the food industry on the world stage, gets less publicity at home. I heard him speak in Vienna at a World Health Organisation ministerial conference on nutrition and non-communicable diseases (heart disease, stroke, diabetes, cancer and lung conditions, most of which are caused or worsened by obesity). His most scathing comments are reserved for what he describes as ultra-processed foods. Yet even that is a misnomer, he said.

'They are formulations and not foods. They are dishes made from foods,' he said.

Even bread which is sold as wholemeal has been processed. 'When people talk about whole bran, it is not whole flour – it is refined,' he said. 'The food industry is trying to reconstruct our food from parts of food and say this is the same or better.' But we were not designed to eat processed foods, which have had nutrients extracted and then sometimes processed back in afterwards, such as vitamins and minerals which may protect you from cancer in the original fruit and vegetables but may not have the same effect as an additive. Vitamin C pills, after all, do not do you as much good as eating oranges. The human race is in the middle of an experiment, he believes.

Monteiro contributed to the Big Food series of articles published in 2012 by the journal *PLOS Medicine*, which was led by Marion Nestle, professor of nutrition at New York University and David Stuckler, senior associate research fellow at Oxford University. Food systems today, dominated by a handful of massive multinational corporations, are not delivering what the world needs, they said.

'Food systems are not driven to deliver optimal human diets but to maximise profits,' wrote Stuckler and Nestle in the opening paper. 'For people living in poverty, this means either exclusion from development (and consequent food insecurity) or eating low-cost, highly processed foods lacking in nutrition and rich in sugar, salt and saturated fats (and consequent overweight and obesity).'

Big Food rules, they said. In the US, the ten largest food companies control over half of all food sales. They are expanding rapidly into the rest of the world and so far control about 15 per cent of the global market. Three quarters of global food sales involve processed foods. More than half of global soft drinks are made by large multinational companies, mainly PepsiCo and Coca-Cola. 'What people eat is increasingly driven by a few multinational food companies,' they wrote. The affluent countries of north America and Europe are now more or less saturated. Pretty much all the growth is now in developing countries.

What is happening in Mexico and other Latin American countries has spread or will spread to other continents as the food and drink industries seek out other markets. India, China and other parts of Asia are huge markets. Africa is on the rise. Obesity follows in the wake.

How deeply entrenched Coca-Cola is in Mexico was evident in Coyoacán, the beautiful former village, now a borough of Mexico City, where the painter Frida Kahlo, partner of Diego Rivera, was born and spent the last years of her life in the 'casa azul' – the blue house. Through the elegant, tree-lined streets, parks, piazzas and pavement cafes I walked, to the traditional covered market. There were stalls selling clothes, jewellery, gifts and every type of fruit and vegetable including an amazing variety of chilli peppers, meat, fish and cheese. In the heart of the market were dozens of red and yellow restaurants and cafes. Every menu board, every refrigerator, every stool was in the red of Coca-Cola. The cooks and waiters all wore yellow T-shirts and red Coca-Cola aprons. Bottles of Coca-Cola were included in the price of many meals. And that was just one small corner of the Coca-Cola empire.

10

SO WHAT CAN WE DO ABOUT IT?

From the fat gradually strangling our organs to the junk food pushed at our children through games on their mobile phones – the more I have looked into the causes and consequences of our weight problems, the more outraged I have become at how little we talk about this and how little is being done to turn the tide.

Nothing happens unless you admit there is a problem. That's the first thing. Denial is a killer. It allows us to sleepwalk into crisis. Who thinks about their weight until they realise their clothes are too tight? And the first initiative we take to deal with that is to move up a size and buy some more. Perhaps we start to worry about our appearance and think about a diet – the sort of 'fix-your-life' fruitarian or fasting or meat and fish diet that the fashion mags credit for the svelte bodies of our favourite actors. And when that fails and more weight piles on, we're in trouble and haunted by feelings of guilt and shame. Each of us is on our own, with scant help beyond advice to 'read the label'. As a society, we're doing hardly more than fiddling at the margins to try to fix a problem that involves all of us and is not to do with sloth or greed but is embedded in the way we live today.

This book has been a journey for me – an exploration of the problem and an attempt to look for ways through it. This is what I have learned.

Everybody says it is complex. That's an excuse for doing nothing or too little. Yes, it is complex, but there are a whole load of things we could try if we had the will. Some of them are for us as individuals and others are for society as a whole. And in my personal view, they would not only make us thinner – but make us happier as well.

You can't turn the clock back, say so many people. That's another excuse for doing nothing. In fact, I think you can. We don't have to return to the paleolithic age, living in caves, hunting, gathering and squatting shivering by a stick fire in our animal skins in the winter. We don't even have to return to the pre-internet, pre-microwave age when women (nearly always women) were slaves to the sink and the stove. There is no need to embrace the bad things about the old days along with the good. We just need to recognise what we have lost and regain it. That's not turning the clock back – it's revival. Young people today do it all the time, rediscovering music from the 70s and 80s. And fashion is cyclical – hemlines go up and down.

What have we lost? For one thing, our sense that eating is a convivial affair, where we sit down and share the occasion with other people. Yes, we do that on a special night out in a restaurant or at a dinner party. But in much of our daily lives, we are grabbing food and eating on the go. Food is fuel to enable us to function. We hardly taste it – and so we buy a chocolate bar or a cake or a packet of sweets to eat mid-morning or mid-afternoon. That's not just about hunger. The snack culture thrives on our disappointment in a breakfast or lunch we hardly noticed because we were running out of the door, on the bus or eating at our desk. Mondelēz can sell chocolate as a little bit of joy because we had a joyless lunch. And what does this habit of rushed convenience food do to our children? A colleague of mine taking the bus was appalled to hear two children on the way to school say to their mother, 'Can we have our breakfast now?' and watch her take two packets of crisps out of her bag. That was their morning routine. It's anecdotal, of course, but there's plenty of evidence of children arriving at school without any breakfast at all or being hyperactive and then later too tired to concentrate after buying an energy drink full of sugar on the way.

So maybe we need more respect for food. We need to factor in time to eat proper meals in the company of others and to digest and to feel satisfied by what we have eaten.

Time. But that's what we don't have in the modern world, people say. Yet how can that be true? We have labour-saving devices, we have fridges, microwaves (nothing wrong with using them to cook real food) and dishwashers. We have supermarkets that take orders online and deliver to the door. And there are any number of cookery books and internet recipes (complete with links to the ingredients to order from your supermarket) that show us how to cook good food quickly, easily and even cheaply.

I would argue we are being duped by those who want to sell us pre-packaged, processed meals, which are full of salt, sugar and saturated fat to try to make up for the absence of fresh ingredients. They may take 10 minutes to heat up. Double that time to 20 minutes and you can cook a really good, simple fresh meal for the whole family in the evening, which will taste so much better. The idea of speed-eating is far more attractive than the reality.

And why can't we bring back family meals as psychologist Suzanne Higgs and, indeed, politician Anna Soubry suggested? If everyone is eating different things at different times, it encourages grazing and snacking and also resistance in children to trying new foods. TV dinners are a disaster because we don't register the amount of food we are consuming. And it's not as if we need to watch anything live any more. Yes, there will be fights around the table as children complain about what's on their plate, but you have good conversations too. And either way, at least you are talking.

What has happened to our eating habits is part of the big social dynamic of the last half century or more. We are each alone. Our community structures and to some extent our families have broken down. Individuals are told they are empowered as a result. You can do what you want, not what others do. It is liberation – or we have been set adrift, depending on your point of view.

That's why I am fascinated by an experiment that started in two small towns in northern France, near Lille, and has since spread to more French towns and other countries. It is an attempt to engage a whole community in efforts to combat the lifestyles that cause obesity.

EPODE (the French acronym for Together Let's Prevent Childhood Obesity) began in Fleurbaix and Laventie in 1992, which between them had 6,600 people at the time. Until 2000, the strategy was all about education in the schools – teaching children about food and cooking, taking them on farm visits and growing fruit and vegetables. After that, the whole community was brought in. This is how it was described by the Dutch nutritionist Martijn Katan in the *New England Journal of Medicine* in 2009: 'Everyone from the mayor to shop owners, schoolteachers, doctors, pharmacists, caterers, restaurant owners, sports associations, the media, scientists, and various branches of town government joined in an effort to encourage children to eat better and move around more. The towns built sporting facilities and playgrounds, mapped out walking itineraries, and hired sports instructors. Families were offered cooking workshops, and families at risk were offered individual counselling.'[1]

It was led by the towns' mayors and an obesity champion, who was appointed locally. These were people with drive and enthusiasm but also profound knowledge of their community. It was back, in effect, to the old days when everybody felt they had a responsibility for bringing up the local children, instead of the hands-off, none-of-my-business attitude we mostly have today, with an underlying fear in big cities that we will get thumped or even stabbed if we say anything. And it appeared to work. By 2005, the prevalence in children had dropped to 8.8 per cent, while in similar neighbouring towns it had risen to 17.8 per cent. It wasn't a rigid scientific trial, so we can't be sure the numbers would not have gone down anyway, but many experts are convinced.

Is the EPODE experience translatable to the UK? It certainly has been taken up in other countries – there are now similar projects in Belgium, Spain, the Netherlands, Greece and Australia, while Mexico is interested. But there are issues. One is that the finance has come from the private sector, including the food companies that are part of the problem – Nestlé and Coca-Cola are among them.

But talking to Carolyn Summerbell, a professor of human nutrition at Durham University and one of the UK's leading obesity experts, it is clear that sponsorship is not the only issue. She was at a meeting with the department of health some years ago to discuss whether an EPODE-type project could be launched in a British town. 'I think there was a feeling that in the UK – and I guess this is rather sad but possibly true – that community spirit, local engagement which is required for the project isn't there and couldn't be resurrected, in that people don't know who lives in the next house, never mind the next street. Communities aren't what they used to be. It's very sad. That could relate to all sorts of projects but it also related to EPODE,' she told me.

'In my dad's day there was the Round Table, there were community groups, even pubs – look at how many of them are closing down now, partly because you can't smoke in them, partly because they are more expensive, partly because you can buy cheaper booze and drink in.'

Those sorts of groups and meeting places, she said, kept people connected. We cannot and will not unplug the internet and shun Facebook and online shopping, but there is a real need to rediscover and reconnect our communities. Wouldn't it be great if some small towns or villages in the UK were to take it upon themselves to try an EPODE-like project in their community? It might even do more to make people happier than help them lose weight.

Thirty years ago and more, when Mrs Thatcher told us there was no such thing as society and that we should be self-reliant and make our own fortune, there may have seemed to be no down-side as consumerism thrived and fast-food outlets sprung up in the high street. Grabbing a bite to eat on the go meant we could work harder. Convenience meals meant we could play harder. The consequences are now highly visible. Food manufacture is the biggest business in the economy. In every town and city we have proliferating cafes and restaurants and supermarkets and convenience stores and snack shops, all competing to persuade us to eat more.

Nobody is going to take away our personal responsibility for our health. Each one of us, as individuals, can make changes in our lives for the better. We can change our diet. We can become more active. We can lose weight. But our chances of long-term success are small without support from those around us and changes in the food and built environment. That's where governments have to come in. Laissez-faire has had its day. Doing nothing is not an option if obesity as a national and a global health problem is to be brought under control.

Oxford University-based nutrition scientist Susan Jebb believes that voluntary reductions by the food industry in the calories and sugar, salt and fat in the food and drinks we buy will improve health. She has to – she heads the government's Responsibility Deal with the food and drink manufacturers, restaurants and supermarkets. And yet her own, personal opinion is that a sugar tax would be a good idea. 'I would like to see a tax on sugary drinks,' she told me as she sipped tea without sugar in one of the many cafes on a street near Waterloo station in London. It would create a differential. If sugar-free drinks were cheaper, some people would opt for those instead. But, she says, 'People are incredibly resistant to the concept of tax.'

Jebb, who fronts most of the government initiatives on obesity, is a pragmatist who works within the constraints imposed by politicians but can clearly see what more needs to be done. 'The Responsibility Deal probably isn't enough – but it is a great deal more than other countries. What gets me out of bed is knowing we are doing not a bad job and better than most,' she said.

'Every single food product carries calories. We really need every single food company to be looking at every single food product in its portfolio and saying, is this as good as it could be?' Instead, as she knows better than anyone, some of the big-brand, big-name companies have signed up to some of the pledges, but not all by any means. And smaller companies and one-off cafes, kebab shops and chippies don't even have it on their radar. It is far from ideal.

Jebb recognises that we, the shoppers out to buy food, are up against unfair odds. 'We have really got to look at the environment and make it easier for people to make the healthy choices or stop undermining their efforts by thrusting the unhealthy options into their line of sight,' she said. We think we are intelligent, sensible, rational human beings who choose what we eat. Wrong, she says. 'The truth is it [that choice] is shaped by the environment way more strongly than we accept.' You take a trolley into the super-market intending to buy meat, vegetables and potatoes and come out with cakes and sweets as well. They were on offer. They certainly looked tempting. 'We get subverted by the environment.'

She is exercised by the displays of junk that are in our eye-line or our children's at supermarkets, noting that food companies pay the stores to get prime positions at the end of aisles. 'What if there were only ever the diet drinks there?' she mused. 'We could do much more. The public, I suspect, will be much more tolerant of interven-tions which shift the balance of how easy or difficult it is [to buy unhealthy food] rather than overt bans.'

For public, read governments afraid of unpopularity and lost votes. I am reminded of the ban on smoking in public places. The Labour government dragged its feet, proposing a partial ban, until public pressure persuaded ministers to allow MPs a free vote in February 2006 – and the full ban went through.

Jebb will continue to try to persuade the companies to make their food and drinks healthier (and in smaller sizes), but at the same time she thinks we all need junk-avoidance skills. Those advertisers and marketing people who shell out for the prime positions for chocolate bars find us very easy prey. They have done their research and know our weaknesses. We need, she said, 'to do much more to help the public to see the impact that the food environment is having on their own choices and their children.' We have not been taught to be suspicious. We need to be given the knowledge and resilience to negotiate our way around the biscuits and chocolate piled high in the supermarket and the cream-loaded pastries in the cafes.

Deborah Cohen of the Rand Institute in California has been working on redesigning supermarkets, so they don't grab attention to the bad food over the good and no sweets are allowed where harassed parents with irritable children are queuing to pay. It just takes away the danger. The Children's Food Campaign in the UK encourages shoppers to hand in red cards at supermarkets where there are unhealthy snacks by the till, saying the store has failed the checkout test. Cohen is also working with food trucks – vans that sell hot fast food in the street – encouraging the families that own them to try more healthy menus.

These sorts of changes to the food environment have to be helpful. We need a respite from the heavily marketed junk that comes in twin packs and BOGOF (buy one get one free) offers.

However, it's the voluntary agreements with industry that are still the flagship initiatives of the governments of market-based economies like the UK and the United States and they are having little real effect. The truth is that fattening junk makes money – a lot of money. We have to ask what would induce multibillion dollar companies with shareholders biting at their heels to cut their profits.

One of the biggest food and drink corporations in the world claims to have seen the light. PepsiCo's chief executive, Indra Nooyi, says she is leading a revolution in the vast snack food and cola company, directing its food scientists and researchers to find new healthy products and improve the ones they already sell. She has sold off some of its less healthy lines and is investing in research into 'better for you' products and ingredients, including natural, low-calorie sweeteners. She says she believes that companies such as hers face decline if they do not respond to the growing concern of consumers about the nutritional value of their food and drink.

The great PepsiCo experiment is worth a closer look, because if Nooyi really can deliver healthier foods, it could impact the diet of billions of people worldwide. Among those who were persuaded by her vision was one of the most respected figures in global public health. To the astonishment of some of his peers, Derek Yach, who had successfully led the World Health Organisation's tobacco control efforts and then fought the food industry over sugar and other nutrients in food, chose to throw in his lot with Nooyi. If anyone was capable of bringing about change in the products that a big snacking corporation sells, he was surely the man.

Yach is a South African public health doctor who enjoys long-distance swimming. He has crossed the Channel, swum the Hudson River and done what is known as the Robben Island double (from Three Anchor Bay in Cape Town to the island and back, which is about 20km). His move from the public sector with WHO to the private sector at PepsiCo (via academia) was a challenge as big as any he had faced. Some of his friends and former colleagues in public health no longer wanted anything to do with him. In some quarters, he was a pariah. Journals would no longer print his articles. But Ricardo Uauy, then president of the International Union of Nutritional Sciences, spoke up for him in the journal *Public Health Nutrition*. 'My position is that Derek is genuine in his motives and he has chosen this job as a new challenge and opportunity to influence the private sector from within. It takes someone like Derek to take on this daunting task, and I propose that we not only give him the benefit of the doubt, but clearly support his efforts and do our best for him to be effective,' he wrote.

Plenty of academics and public health experts have taken industry money to sit on advisory boards. Indeed, Yach points out that his former boss at the WHO, Director-General Gro Harlem Brundtland, once prime minister of Norway, was on PepsiCo's advisory board when he arrived, to the horror of some of Norway's newspapers. But Yach went to PepsiCo not to advise but in order to try to make things happen from within.

Indra Nooyi called, out of the blue, a month before she became CEO, he told me when we met in London in 2013. 'She invited me in and painted a vision of what she wanted to do,' he said. 'There was no talk about a job. It was a strange day. So here I am at PepsiCo headquarters, she knows exactly my background and she really sketched out the fact that it's inevitable that change has to come to the food sector. She was the one, as the chief financial officer, who sold off Taco Bell, Kentucky Fried Chicken and Pizza Hut [she spun them off into the separate company, Yum!, in 1997]. And she was the chief financial officer who acquired Tropicana, Gatorade and Quaker. Whereas you may worry about Gatorade, Quaker and Trop were at the time the "halo" food companies in the US. So if I had to have proof that she was serious, this was absolute proof. She said what she really wanted was somebody who was going to be as critical internally as I had been outside and we've really got to bring about the change. I was kind of shocked. I didn't know what to do.'

If you've ever met Indra, said Yach, you will know that she doesn't ask – she tells you what you will be doing for her. It was not an interview, but the start of his new job.

He spent five years there and said he gave himself a 65 per cent success rating by the end of it. 'What we never anticipated was the recession. What I never knew was the power of consumer demand. They just want this unhealthy stuff,' he said.

'I still don't think that the marketing people really know how to turn on the kind of messages to sell healthier things that often cost marginally more and come with less volume than the cheap easy stuff – sodas and chips and things. I've been intrigued ever since to understand.

'You've got this divergence now in the US between a large group calling for healthy food – the most affluent usually in the country, who can afford healthier things – and the fact that Twinkies, surely the unhealthiest product on the planet, went into bankruptcy and got salvaged by investors to put Twinkies back on the market. You'd have thought the demand for Twinkies was dead but clearly it isn't and it's booming.

'It's a white creamy thing in a type of synthetic bread which has a shelf life of about a decade. It's pure processed junk. I've even seen a chocolate-covered Twinkie and a deep-fried Twinkie. It's like a cult thing. They are a cult thing for unhealthy eating in America – but much beloved.'

But demand is also high for sushi, he reflected, which is one of the healthiest foods anyone can eat. 'Sushi has exploded and nobody seems to be able to tell me why,' he said.

There are unexpected trends. Sushi is, of course, not a brand but a type of food, which people are clearly getting a taste for. It comes packaged for lunchtime eating or snacks. The Twinkie cult owes more to old habits and our appetite for decades now for fat and sugar. The efforts of the marketing men and women will not change our preferences overnight, but the problem at PepsiCo, it appeared, was – in the end – that there was a limit to how much they were prepared to try. Money shouts loudest. There may have been a willingness at the very top to launch new healthy ranges, but they were always going to be dumped if they did not make big profits. Yach spoke of a trip to Brazil to investigate the possibility of a 'righteous food' programme, involving the marketing of very nutritious tropical fruits. The idea had emerged from a discussion years before with Geoffrey Cannon, a food and nutrition expert who was working as an adviser to the Brazilian government and who joined Yach and a PepsiCo marketing man on the exploratory trip.

'The trip was frustrating, because the marketing executive, who kept on telling me "here's the thing", was not interested in righteousness,' wrote Cannon five years afterwards in a blog in December 2012.[2] 'He also kept on talking about "low-hanging fruit", a metaphor here applied to actual fruit, which meant raw material that could be branded and on sale the next year.'

The marketing man was unenthused. The plan came to nothing. 'Unfortunately, internally the traction for that wasn't there because it didn't meet the business models,' said Yach.

In the UK, there was Planet Lunch, the brainwave of a forward-thinking PepsiCo executive who wanted to sell healthy snack boxes for children. He talked with the Food Standards Authority and ensured the snack boxes met its strict nutrition requirements. 'The product got launched and was run in test markets but the price was too high,' said Yach. 'In time it probably would have made it, but [...] PepsiCo is such a large company that success means making it to half a billion or a billion-dollar revenue. If you've got 22 brands worth a billion dollars a year each, to make it to that level you've got to be a blockbuster over-night or you must get killed. I saw many of what struck me, as a health person, as being great products dying because the business model couldn't work.'

On the positive side, there was Sabra Hummus, which is 50 per cent owned by PepsiCo, Müller yoghurt, Tropicana 50, which is a lower-calorie version of the juice drink, and Diet Mountain Dew, which actually hit the billion-dollar mark. 'So there are these examples of good successes, but there are not as many as you'd want.'

Yach left PepsiCo after five years for several reasons. He had been invited to lead the US expansion of a South African company engaged in health promotion – he is now director of the Vitality Institute in New York. He also felt he had achieved a certain amount, particularly on the R&D agenda and setting nutritional standards for the company to work towards in new products. Indra had wanted him to set quantifiable goals, he said. Those in WHO and campaign groups who said 'you cannot expect to trust industry to say anything unless they can show the numbers' were absolutely right. 'So we set the [PepsiCo] American targets for salt, sugar, fats – not only for that but goals were set for withdrawing full-calorie sodas from schools around the world.' There were more targets for new fruits, vegetables, grains, and nuts-based products, to encourage investment in those lines. The next few years would be harder, he thought, not least because of the recession. His decision to go was not, he said, in any way connected with pressure on Indra Nooyi to change tack when PepsiCo's share price fell and Coca-Cola surged ahead. Nor did he leave because he was disenchanted with the work.

Nooyi wanted him because he was a critic of the food industry, according to Uauy, who wrote that she told him: 'We have asked Derek to change this company; in five years we want to have most of our product line meet the international standards supporting life-long health … if he fails we fail.'

Yach could not be said to have failed but nor was the venture an overwhelming success. He achieved some things, but the issues of billion-dollar sales and share prices remain after his departure, and no doubt will do after Nooyi's. The insight he gives us into the global food industry suggests that profits will always get in the way of the health agenda. We cannot rely on the reformulation of essentially unhealthy and unnecessary foods to get us out of this crisis.

Yach still sounds like a man from WHO. When I asked about sports sponsorship, he linked fast food firmly with tobacco, which he played a leading part years ago in getting banned from advertising at the Olympics. 'You would never have thought in the beginning of the 1990s that tobacco sponsorship of sport would become unacceptable and now alcohol and some of the fast-food products are clearly next,' he said.

He even said that greater government intervention would be good for the industry. 'I think for the food companies, for those looking to the future, it's also in their best interests to have government far more aggressive about the value of fruits and vegetables and nuts and grains and making it far more difficult for the marketing of products that are most associated with unhealthy diets to be available, by encouraging the healthier ones.

'I can't imagine broccoli becoming a major sponsor of the Olympics in the short term but why not, long term? Why wouldn't you have Birds Eye with their frozen vegetables? It sounds crazy but ask kids today – can you imagine that Marlboro was sponsoring the Olympics? They look at you as if you are crazy, but that was the case.'

Many public health campaigners think it is a mistake to try to do deals with industry. 'I don't know what he was thinking,' said Marion Nestle, professor of nutrition at New York University, of Yach, whom she used to consider 'a public health hero' at WHO. 'If you want to advise people to be healthier, they have to eat less of these products. That's very bad for business. That's the problem.'

Geoffrey Cannon says that the industry is much bigger and more hydra-headed than people imagine. Rather than the 'food and drink industry', we should be talking about 'food and drink transnational manufacturers, distributors, retailers and caterers', he said. 'They work as a pack. When they are threatened with any kind of regulation or supervision from government, they all gang together. These alliances that very readily persuade the UN and national governments that, for example, voluntary food labelling is where it's at, prove that the food and drink transnationals are not competitive. When the chips are down, they work together.'

We cannot rely on the food and drink industry to promote broccoli over biscuits or even frozen peas over pasties. It is not in their interests. These are not health companies, but profit-making processed food giants. They don't grow food – they engineer it and mass-produce it in factories.

So governments and international organisations have got to stop pretending the companies will sort this out and take obesity far more seriously. It is not about a few sad individuals who have to be evacuated from their homes by the fire brigade. Firstly we need education and information – not denial. That starts with the youngest. Compulsory cooking lessons and nutrition education in schools for all children is a great move. So are bans on vending machines containing sweets and colas in schools. But voluntary agreements, for instance on traffic light labelling on the front of packs, with red lights for foods high in salt, fat or sugar, are just not enough. The Children's Food Campaign has a 'wall of shame', where it posts details of the companies that are dragging their feet or plain refusing to co-operate. They point the finger at the big American food companies: 'It's not just General Mills [which owns Nestlé breakfast cereals]. There seems to be a common theme emerging amongst those who have made it onto our labelling wall of shame. Heinz, Coca-Cola, Kellogg's (and even Cadbury via Mondelēz) are all American-owned corporations. Could it be that the US headquarters of these companies are dragging their feet (or just being plain obstructionist) about signing up their UK brands to the new labelling scheme? If that is indeed the case, why should America – years behind the UK and Europe in terms of most of its health and nutrition policies, and infamous for its well-financed and (sadly) hugely effective corporate food lobby – be dictating what happens on our supermarket shelves here? Why should they be preventing millions of British consumers from having the best nutritional advice on products?'

These are some of the vast corporations that are head-quartered in the US, but effectively run the food systems of the entire globe. It is not in their interests to set a prece-dent in the UK by slapping warning signs on their cereals, biscuits and sweets, as we do on packets of cigarettes. That would make the parallel between junk food and tobacco increasingly apparent.

That is why there has been intense lobbying going on in Latin America, where civil society campaigners and public health experts have taken on food labelling and marketing to children and succeeded in persuading politicians to legislate. The schemes in Chile, Peru and Ecuador are not voluntary agreements with food and drinks manufacturers – they are legally binding. Chile, for instance, is requiring a warning label covering 10 per cent of the packet of any food that is high in either salt or saturated fat or sugar. It has also passed restrictions on marketing to children. The food industry has been fighting this overtly and covertly since it was first proposed, claiming it will damage trade and is an infringement of individual rights. The bill was passed in the Chilean Senate in July 2012, but nobody knows when it will be implemented, because of the opposition.

'Governments see the rising tsunami of obesity flooding over their countries, but as soon as they put up serious policies to create healthier food environments they get hammered by the food industry,' said Professor Barry Popkin from the University of Carolina at the launch of the Bellagio Declaration by public health experts in the summer of 2013. The declaration called on the WHO to establish norms for the way governments and food and drinks companies do business, 'so that partnerships are not detrimental to nutrition goals'.

So Latin America is teaching us the way to go. The outcome of the sweetened soft drinks tax that has been passed by Mexico's Congress will be closely watched.

The UK should and could embrace food taxes too, to make unhealthy food comparatively more expensive than food that is unquestionably good for us. At the moment, junk food appears cheap and fresh fruit and vegetables seem expensive. Mike Rayner, director of the British Heart Foundation Health Promotion Research Group, which is part of the Nuffield Department of Population Health at Oxford University, is the chief advocate of food taxes in the UK. He is also vice chair of Sustain and chair of the Children's Food Campaign, which is lobbying specifically for a sugary drinks tax. Rayner thinks there is beginning to be a climate of opinion in the UK in which higher taxes on unhealthy food and drink, to change this imbalance, might be possible.

'Obviously I'm a proponent of taxing more than just sugary drinks. I think the VAT system should be reformed in line with health goals. But as a first measure we were proposing, and I think people have come behind this, the idea of taxing sugary drinks,' he told me.

He cites experiments in some European countries. In 2011, the Danes brought in duty on saturated fat, which infuriated the butter and bacon industries and was withdrawn after a political storm a year later. However, it was, Rayner says, a fascinating experiment that could yield very useful scientific data.

'What's interesting from a researcher's point of view is that we have a period when it wasn't there, a year when it was there and now a period when it wasn't there, so we'll be able to see changes in consumption patterns and possibly even changes in health effects like blood cholesterol levels – the consequences of that tax. So from a research point of view it's a dream,' he said.

The tax had a bad press and has been thrown at health campaigners ever since by the food industry as an example of why food taxes won't work. It was badly thought out, invented by the Treasury to raise money, so it was not health-inspired. Stories circulated that Danes were crossing the border in their cars and loading up with cheaper meat and dairy foods. Health campaigners allege the tales that ran in the papers were industry-inspired. Food industry sources around the world say the tax was a failure. Rayner and others say there is evidence it was a success. 'We're beginning to get the preliminary results of the actual tax … and it did seem to have quite a significant effect on saturated fat levels or butter consumption and other things in Denmark,' he said. France introduced a tax of 7 cents per litre of soft drink in December 2011, although in response to industry lobbying, it was imposed on all soft drinks and did not stigmatise those with high sugar content. That brought sales down by 4 per cent.

Taxes and subsidies to adjust the food supply are far from new. Many argue that a large part of the problem we have today was caused by government subsidies in the country that more than any is identified with the free market – the United States. The subsidies for corn and other 'white' crops brought in decades ago to protect America's farmers have resulted in huge surpluses of the wrong sort of food, as is very obvious in Mississippi. If there are to be any subsidies, they should now be switched to the fresh foods that are good for us, encouraging farmers to grow more of them and all of us to eat them as the prices come down.

Even if the government will not act to save us from ourselves, they have to protect children. Passive smoking finally nailed tobacco. It was the evidence that non-smokers were in danger of disease by inhaling other people's cigarette fumes that spurred the government on to the ban on smoking in public places. It is getting ever harder for governments to dodge the argument that the food environment is harming children.

Psychology professor Jane Ogden, who treats people with such morbid obesity that they cannot get out of a wheelchair, thinks we are getting to a point where the personal responsibility argument just will not hold. Passive smoking she describes as 'the tipping point where society said, "Hold on a minute – I'm not going to be quite so libertarian with you and say you can do what you like to yourself because I don't like it in my world." I think with obesity perhaps the same tipping point will come when it starts to be seen that the next generation is just following in their parents' footsteps and that child obesity is a form of child abuse, really. OK, somebody can have a BMI of 40 if they want to, but if they have a kid then they also are fat before the age of 10. That really isn't acceptable any longer.'

And the huge financial burden on the NHS may eventually force ministers into more action. 'I think the government has to be much more nanny state around the obesogenic environment in terms of policing the food industry, taxing snack food, taxing fizzy drinks, banning fizzy drinks, banning sugary foods and not just in school dinners but also in work canteens and hospital food. Every kind of food provision that is out there has to be much more controlled by the government. Then they have to put money into cycle paths and street lighting and they have to redesign their cities so they have walking areas and it makes it much more easy for people to be physically active.'

But she says she is thankful she is not prime minister, because she can see the other side of her own argument. 'I do believe all that, but then there is the libertarian in me which says, does that mean they ban Cheesy Wotsits? I mean, my children sometimes have Cheesy Wotsits, but my children are perfectly thin because they don't have them all the time. It is about that conversation. Is that what it means – do we ban Cheesy Wotsits so children only have healthy food? Because the problem with food is that it isn't like cigarettes. Cigarettes are bad per se. Foods are only sort of bad if you have too many of them – apart probably from fizzy drinks which I think are evil.' She laughed. 'You can ban fizzy drinks – I think that's OK.'

Maybe, says Jane Wardle, at UCL's behavioural research centre, we can one day enlist new technology to our aid. She thinks there are some people who find it very much harder to avoid the calorie-dense food environment around us than others. They are genetically primed to put on weight when there is abundant food, she believes, unlike the hunters among us who had to be lean so they could move fast to catch their prey. Those are the people who need extra help in the food-rich modern age. It may be possible to give them cognitive training, so that they can avoid the food cues all around us.

Or, she said, maybe Google will invent some glasses to screen out burgers. They could deliver messages such as 'no – you can have one later but not now!' In fact, she's serious. 'It seems to me that technology will offer us options and maybe there can also be training kind of things. That's just assuming the environment is not going to change and I believe we can't put the genie back in the bottle. We can make crisps cost more, but it's a bit of a drop in the ocean compared with what's happened.'

While Google is working on it and the advertising and promotions are still besieging us, what is the individual to do who may be one of those whom Jane Wardle says are genetically challenged and seem to pile on weight while their luckier friends stay thin? They may not have a very accurate satiety mechanism, she says. They can eat and eat without feeling too full to stop. It's tricky, she says, because people assume they will feel full when their body has had enough. 'You have to say to them, actually, you probably don't, so you might need to use a super-measurement approach to eating. So you might actually need to weigh your cornflakes,' she said. She and colleagues spend a lot of time encouraging people to weigh and measure everything, or buy pre-packed portions, so they know exactly how much they are eating. The fact is that it's easy to under-estimate. An obese person may eat only 300 or 500 calories more than somebody of normal weight in a day. That may amount to no more than a bit extra here and a slightly larger portion there. 'Most obese people will tell you that they don't even see themselves as over-eating and they cry and say, "I don't understand it – I'm eating the same as everybody else, so why am I like this?"' she said. One day there may be a computer chip to attach to your teeth that will count the calories for you or, more likely, drugs that will make you feel full – but not yet.

For people to realise they have a problem that is affecting or will affect their health, there has to be more openness about the harm that obesity does. Jebb thinks the GPs need to tell it as it is. 'I think we are a bit too reticent about telling people they should be going on a diet. A lot of my colleagues are very anxious about it,' she said.

She knows that many diets fail – or rather, she adds, many people who try to diet fail to lose weight and keep it off. But, she says, research shows that on average, it takes people five years to regain all the weight they lost when they were dieting. Jebb, who has done a lot of work with

Weight Watchers, is not condoning fasting or fad diet regimes, she says, but she could see an argument for people dieting to lose maybe 5 per cent of their weight every five years. Obesity is a chronic condition, she says, and people put on weight anyway as they get older. Perhaps we should remember that and accept that we can't just lose enough to be free of it for the rest of our lives.

But I think there is still a huge issue around the way commercial diets are promoted to us. This is the only talk most of us hear about tackling excess weight and it is at best misleading and, at worst, plain cynical. Commercial diets that promise a new, slimline and entrancing body within a few months – with the inbuilt assumption that the regime will come to an end at that time and that, like Cinderella, you will live happily ever after with your handsome (thin) prince – need to be consigned to the dustbin. 'Diet' has two meanings in the Oxford dictionary. The second is: 'a special course of food to which a person restricts themselves, either to lose weight or for medical reasons'. The first is: 'the kinds of food that a person, animal, or community habitually eats'. Exactly. We need a change of emphasis. We need to talk not about 'a diet' but about 'our diet', not about restricting calories but about habitually eating well.

Robert Lustig, author of *Fat Chance: The Bitter Truth About Sugar*, puts it succinctly in three words. Eat real food. Carlos Monteiro in Brazil, scourge of 'ultra-processed food', would agree. If we could all go back to the raw ingredients – fresh fruit and vegetables, fish and chicken – and cook it for ourselves, a large part of the problem would be sorted. But that may take skills we don't have and, as things stand, it may be (or appear to be) a more expensive option for most people. That's why teaching children about food and cooking in schools is so important.

We need to know whether the food we buy is what we think it is. Tests from a public laboratory in West Yorkshire revealed that more than a third of products were not what they claimed to be or were mislabelled in some way. Shocking results published in February 2014 show that we are being sold mozzarella that is less than half real cheese, ham on pizzas that is either poultry or 'meat emulsion', while a herbal slimming tea was neither herb nor tea but glucose powder laced with an obesity drug at 13 times the normal dose.[3] And what are we to make of 'pink slime'? This is the meat equivalent of the chicken nugget – carcass trimmings that are 'warmed, centrifuged to remove the fat, treated with ammonium hydroxide gas to kill pathogens and compressed into blocks that are frozen for later use', according to Marion Nestle at New York University. The meat industry in the United States calls it 'lean finely textured beef' and it is approved for human consumption by the United States Department of Agriculture (USDA). The pejorative 'pink slime', apparently used for years, is uncalled for, says the meat industry. Beef Products Inc, the main producer, which sued ABC News over negative stories about 'pink slime', says that LFTB is highly nutritious and up to 97 per cent lean beef.

Of course, education alone isn't the answer. We might decide we're happy with what we're being sold, even if we know what's in it. Jamie Oliver's experiment, making chicken nuggets out of leftover chicken parts in front of schoolchildren, did not have the result he expected. The kids ate them anyway.

Ian Campbell, Nottinghamshire GP and anti-obesity expert, says eating well has to be made easier for people, as well as cheaper. It is human nature to choose the easy option, he says, just as we always take a shortcut across grass, carving a muddy track, rather than stick to the longer, winding tarmac path. 'The reason why all our great efforts to help people to lose weight don't work is because ultimately it's still easier, for a hundred different reasons, to eat unhealthily than it is to eat healthily and it's easier to be inactive than it is to be active. Ultimately people take the easy option. Until we make healthy choices attractive and easier, people will continue to make bad choices,' he said. Celebrity chefs may give people the wrong idea. It doesn't have to be expensive or complicated. 'Cooking is very simple,' he said.

We also need to recognise that processed food is not as nice as a freshly home-cooked meal. 'Getting that message across starts at school and works its way up, I think,' Campbell said.

And of course we need to be more physically active. Like diets, gym membership works for most people only in the short-term and it is very expensive. We need to build physical activity, which doesn't have to mean rowing machines and treadmills, into our lives. It means going for walks, cycling, gardening, kicking a ball in the park, swimming at the weekends, leaving the car behind some days and just getting up and moving away from the desk during working hours. Local authorities need to turn our towns into more active places by building cycle lanes and footpaths, putting in better street lighting, building public spaces and parks where people can go to meet and walk and improving public transport so people leave their cars at home. They should also provide safe playgrounds for children, street cleaning and pedestrian crossings. Office buildings should have signs to the stairs, showers and secure bike racks. None of this is outrageous. All of these things and more are recommended by NICE in the UK, after teams of experts investigated the evidence for what works and what does not. It won't happen quickly, because no town has the money for such a transformation, but each time planning permission is granted for a block of flats and whenever land is developed, councils need to require that the NICE guidance is followed.

Food and drinks companies, who push hard on sport and exercise as the solution to obesity so that we won't think curbing their advertising spend might help, don't often admit that even gym sessions won't help us lose very much weight. If we are taking in just 300 extra calories a day, we will need to spend more than 45 minutes doing aerobics to burn that off, according to Coca-Cola's own 'Work It Out' calculator. That is to keep our weight stable. If we want to lose weight, we will have to increase the time. Very few of us do anything like that much strenuous exercise on a daily basis.

But physical activity is hugely important because it makes us fitter and healthier even if we are overweight. And it makes us happier. The body releases chemicals called endorphins when we are physically active, which relieve stress, improve our mood and boost our self-esteem. It is well known that exercise helps lift depression.

And less stressed, less depressed, happier people are less likely to resort to food to cheer themselves up or to use it as a crutch against emotional distress and disappointment. We are more likely to wait until we are hungry to eat because, if we are happy, we have other things to think about besides food. A healthy mind is essential for a healthy body, as the old saying goes. The World Health Organisation defines health as 'a state of complete physical, mental and social wellbeing and not merely the absence of disease or infirmity'. Looking at obesity as merely a physical issue, to be sorted out by dieting, will not help control this epidemic. It is far more complex. It is about the way we live today – the social and the built environment – and how we feel about ourselves and our lives. Only if we consider all these things, will we realistically be able to do something about the shape we're in.

ACKNOWLEDGMENTS

I'd like to thank all those who helped and supported me in writing this book. I am especially grateful to Laura Hassan, my brilliant editor at Guardian Faber; Sara Montgomery and Julian Loose, who decided to back the concept; Alex Kirby, for the excellent jacket design; and Lindsay Davies, Andy Armitage, Anna Pallai and John Grindrod, for their enthusiasm and hard work. The book would not have got past first base without my amazing agent, Kate Shaw. Thanks also to Dan Sabbagh, *Guardian* Home Editor, for giving me time to work on some of the stories.

I owe a great deal to all the academics and public health experts fighting the obesity epidemic, who were extremely generous with their time and their knowledge. I cannot name them all here, but Philip James and Simon Capewell were particularly supportive of this project. I also want to thank Rebecca Berner of El Poder del Consumidor, who is a phenomenon and enabled me to learn far more than I could possibly have hoped without her when I visited Mexico. I am also very grateful indeed for the frankness and courage of those people who were willing to tell me their own personal stories.

And finally, thanks to Peter, Katie and Emily Hooley for their unfailing love and support.

ENDNOTES

Chapter 1: We are all in denial

1) A systematic review in 2010 by scientists at Queen's University, Toronto, Canada, estimated that obesity was eating up between 0.7 per cent (in France) and 2.8 per cent (in the USA) of a country's annual total health spending.

2) Johnson et al, 'Changing perceptions of weight in Great Britain', *British Medical Journal*, 2008.

3) Figures are from the Health Survey for England 2007–2010, which also showed that the second most affluent group of men have the highest obesity levels, at 26.7 per cent, while the worst off average 25.5 per cent. Accessed from the National Obesity Observatory (now Public Health England).

4) According to a paper by Angus Nicholl et al from the Public Health Laboratory Service in a study published in the journal *Sexually Transmitted Infections* in 2001.

5) Cameron went on to say: 'We talk about people being "at risk of obesity" instead of talking about people who eat too much and take too little exercise. We talk about people being at risk of poverty, or social exclusion; it's as if these things – obesity, alcohol abuse, drug addiction – are purely external events like a plague or bad weather. Of course, circumstances – where you are born, your neighbourhood, your school, and the choices your parents make – have a huge impact. But social problems are often the consequence of the choices that people make.'

Chapter 2: Sugar, fat and alcohol – a deadly trio?

1) There is 34.6g of sugar in a standard 58g Mars Bar.

2) IASO collected data from the UK food purchase surveys and UN Food and Agriculture Organisation Food Balance Sheets.

3) Not everyone agrees with Volkow's findings. Other scientists, particularly those with links to the food and drink industry, dismiss the addiction theory, saying it is effectively used as an excuse for people whose eating behaviours are out of control.

4) The British Soft Drink Association says 61 per cent of the nearly 227 litres of all soft drinks that each person drank in the UK in 2012 had no added sugar. But that category of 'no added sugar' includes fruit juice and smoothies.

5) COMA (the committee on medical aspects of food policy), 'Dietary reference values for food energy and nutrients for the United Kingdom', published by the Department of Health, 1991, responding to evidence primarily about tooth decay.

6) Weichselbaum, E, 'Is sugar really that bad for you?', *Nutrition Bulletin*, 11 May 2012, published by the British Nutrition Foundation.

7) It rested its case on reviews by the German Nutrition Society in 2012 and the European Food Safety Authority (EFSA) in 2010.

8) Formerly the Sugar Bureau.

9) The World Sugar Research Organisation is an international body funded by Coca-Cola and the sugar manufacturers of 30 countries. They claim they are 'committed to upholding the fundamental principles of science and to relying solely on objective science in its programmes'.

Chapter 3: All-day eating

1) The paper said: 'With no specific guidance on snacking in the UK, many may be unclear about the effects of snacking on health and the best food and drink choices to make if eating between meals ... The so-called obesity epidemic appears to have coincided with a change in eating patterns and, in some countries, a possible increase in the intake of snacks. Whether changes in eating patterns, an increase in eating or snacking frequency and/or changes in the nutrient composition of snacks have specifically contributed to this obesity trend remains questionable, despite scientific research interest in the field for a number of decades ... for some individuals, including young children, snacking may have a positive rather than negative impact on health and should not be discouraged on a population-wide basis. Depending on food choice, snacks and increased meal frequency could contribute to a healthy energy and nutrient intake and may have metabolic and cognitive benefits. However, evidence remains inconsistent and further good-quality studies are needed in this field.'

Chapter 4: The fattest towns in Britain

1) In the 2012 update, the National Obesity Observatory (now part of Public Health England), published figures on obesity and overweight combined, which they called 'excess weight'. Tamworth was 25th in the country, on 70.7 per cent. Gateshead was down at 239th place (out of 327), on 61.9 per cent. The highest rate – 75.9 per cent – was in Copeland, Cumbria.

2) The average household income in the town in 2010 was £36,800, but the average income range ran from £27,000 in Glascote ward to £43,700 in affluent Trinity.

3) Figures are taken from the 2008 Lifestyle Survey of NHS South of Tyne and Wear.

Chapter 5: So where's the harm?

1) Dr Sharma's Obesity Notes (www.drsharma.ca/class-1-obesity-dont-worry-be-happy.html).

2) See for instance Wagner, B et al, 'Extreme obesity is associated with suicidal behavior and suicide attempts in adults: results of a population-based representative sample', *Depression and Anxiety*, October 2013.

3) Rudd Report, *Weight Bias: A Social Justice Issue*, 2012.

4) Muennig, P et al, 'I think therefore I am: perceived ideal weight as a determinant of health', *American Journal of Public Health*, March 2008.

5) Abramson, J, 'Should people at low risk of cardiovascular disease take a statin?', *British Medical Journal*, October 2013.

Chapter 6: The diets don't work

1) *The Men Who Made Us Thin*, BBC2, 2013.

2) Interviewed on BBC Radio 4's *Start the Week*, 20 January 2014.

3) Leibel, RL, Rosenbaum, M, and Hirsch, J, 'Changes in energy expenditure resulting from altered body weight', *New England Medical Journal*, 1995.

4) *Financial Times*, 17 January 2014.

Chapter 7: Child abuse?

1) The BBC afterwards surveyed 50 consultant paediatricians, who said that obesity had been a factor in 20 child protection cases in the previous year. It was not necessarily the only reason, but it was one of the factors being taken into account when judgment was made on the safety of a child's home.

2) Perez-Pastor, E at al, 'Assortative weight gain in mother-daughter and father-son pairs: an emerging source of childhood obesity', *International Journal of Obesity*, July 2009.
3) Source: *Diabetes in the UK 2012: Key Statistics*, Diabetes UK. The very first cases in the UK were detected in 2000 among young girls of Indian, Pakistani or Arabic origin. Two years later, the disease was diagnosed in white adolescents too.
4) Obesity is not measured in the same way in children as in adults. BMI in children is based on growth charts, which show the weight a child should have reached not only for his or her height but compared to other children of their age.
5) Jeffery, AN et al, 'Parents' awareness of overweight in themselves and their children' (EarlyBird 21), *British Medical Journal*, 2005.
6) Mattison, J et al, 'Impact of calorie restriction on health and survival in rhesus monkeys from the NIA study', *Nature*, September 2012.
7) *Marketing of Foods High in Fat, Salt and Sugar to Children: update 2012–2013*, WHO Europe.
8) Data from 2011 showed that 65 per cent of children aged between five and seven in the UK used the internet on computers in their home, which rose to 85 per cent of children aged eight to 11. Many children had mobile phones – one in eight aged eight to 11 and one in 50 aged five to seven in the UK owned a smartphone.
9) *Fast Food Facts 2013*, Yale Rudd Center.
10) The spokesman continued: 'Our sponsorship of sporting events highlights our commitment to making a positive difference in all the communities we serve. We care about people's wellbeing and want to make a positive difference in their lives, both physically and emotionally. We also aspire to help people lead active healthy lifestyles through the beverage options we produce, the nutritional information we provide and our support of programmes that encourage active, healthy living.'

Chapter 8: America's big problem

1) The Centers for Disease Control reported Louisiana had 34.7 per cent obesity to Mississippi's 34.6 per cent.
2) The fact Johnson cites is taken from a study in the *New England Journal of Medicine* in March 2005 by SJ Olshansky et al, which for the first time published data showing the damage to life expectancy likely to be caused by the obesity epidemic. The Robert Wood Johnson Foundation disseminated the message that this could be the first generation of children to live sicker and die younger than their parents.

3) Source: Pomeranz, J and Rutkow, L, 'Efforts to immunize food manufacturers from obesity-related lawsuits: a challenge for public health', City University of New York-based *Corporations and Health Watch*, August 2011.
4) Brownell, K, 'Personal responsibility and obesity', *Health Affairs*, 2010.
5) These guidelines are taken from the food industry's own revised Children's Food and Beverage Advertising Initiative nutrition standards or the National Restaurant Association's Kids LiveWell standards.
6) Brownell & Frieden, 'Ounces of Prevention', *New England Journal of Medicine*, 2009. Kelly Brownell is first credited with the idea as early as 1994.

Chapter 9: Mexicoke

1) Nestlé's response to a story about the controversy in the *British Medical Journal* was that it aimed to help families eat better and that the women it trained would not be tied to using its own products. Quaker Mexico was happy that its products would be nutritious and affordable.

Chapter 10: So what can we do about it?

1) Katan, M, editorial, 'Weight-loss diets for the prevention and treatment of obesity', *New England Journal of Medicine*, February 2009.
2) Geoffrey Cannon blogs for the World Public Health Nutrition Association.
3) Lawrence, F, 'Fake-food scandal revealed as tests show third of products mislabelled', *Guardian*, 8 February 2014.

BIBLIOGRAPHY

Books

Baggini, Julian, *The Virtues of the Table: How to Eat and Think*, Granta, 2014

Cohen, Deborah, *A Big Fat Crisis: The Hidden Forces Behind the Obesity Epidemic and How We Can End It*, Nation Books, 2014

Hastings, Gerard, *The Marketing Matrix: How the Corporation Gets Its Power – and How We Can Reclaim It*, Routledge, 2012

James, Philip, 'Obesity', *Oxford Textbook of Public Health*, 5th edition, Oxford University Press, 2011

Lustig, Robert, *Fat Chance: The Hidden Truth About Sugar, Obesity and Disease*, Fourth Estate, 2014

Nestle, Marion, *Food Politics: How the Food Industry Influences Nutrition and Health*, University of California Press, June 2013

Ogden, Jane, *The Psychology of Eating: From Healthy to Disordered Behaviour*, Wiley Blackwell, 2010

Ogden, Jane, *The Good Parenting Food Guide: Managing What Children Eat Without Making Food a Problem*, Wiley Blackwell, 2014

Orbach, Susie, *Fat is a Feminist Issue*, Arrow, first edition 1978

Orbach, Susie, *Bodies*, Profile, 2010

Orbach, Susie, *On Eating: Change Your Eating, Change Your Life*, Penguin, 2002

Yudkin, John, *Pure, White and Deadly: How Sugar Is Killing Us and What We Can Do to Stop It*, Penguin, first edition 1972

Medical reports

Academy of Medical Royal Colleges, *Measuring Up: The Medical Profession's Prescription for the Nation's Obesity Crisis*, February 2013

European Heart Network, *Diet, Physical Activity and Cardiovascular Disease Prevention*, November 2011

Foresight, *Tackling Obesities: Future Choices*, Government Office for Science, October 2007

Institute for Health Metrics and Evaluation, *Global Burden of Diseases, Injuries, and Risk Factors Study*, 2010

Keys, Ancel, *Seven Countries: A Multivariate Analysis of Death and Coronary Heart Disease*, Harvard University Press, 1980

Royal College of Physicians, *Action on Obesity: Comprehensive Care for All*, January 2013

Rudd Report, *Weight Bias: A Social Justice Issue*, Yale Rudd Center, 2012

Trust for America's Health and the Robert Wood Johnson Foundation, *F as in Fat: How Obesity Threatens America's Future*, September 2012

World Health Organisation, *Diet, Nutrition and the Prevention of Chronic Disease*, 2003

Scientific papers and articles in journals

Abramson, J, 'Should people at low risk of cardiovascular disease take a statin?', *British Medical Journal*, October 2013

Blom, Wendy et al, 'Effects of 15-d repeated consumption of *Hoodia gordonii* purified extract on safety, ad libitum energy intake, and body weight in healthy, overweight women: a randomized controlled trial', *American Journal of Clinical Nutrition*, October 2011

Bray, George, and Popkin, Barry, 'Calorie-sweetened beverages and fructose: what have we learned 10 years later', *Paediatric Obesity*, August 2013

Brownell, Kelly, 'Personal responsibility and obesity: a constructive approach to a controversial issue', *Health Affairs*, March 2010

Brownell, Kelly D, and Frieden, Thomas R, 'Ounces of Prevention: The Public Policy Case for Taxes on Sugared Beverages', *New England Journal of Medicine*, April 2009

Cohen, Deborah A and Babey, Susan H, 'Candy at the cash register – a risk factor for obesity and chronic disease', *New England Journal of Medicine*, 2012

Cohen, Deborah A and Farley, Thomas, 'Eating as an automatic behaviour', *Preventing Chronic Disease*, 2008

deShazo, Richard D, Bigler, Steven, Baldwin Skipworth, Leigh, 'The autopsy of chicken nuggets reads "Chicken Little"', *American Journal of Medicine*, November 2013

Duffey, Kiyah and Popkin, Barry, 'Energy density, portion size, and eating occasions: contributions to increased energy intake in the United States, 1977–2006', *PLOS Medicine*, June 2011

Flegal, Katherine et al, 'Association of all-cause mortality with overweight and obesity using standard body mass index categories: a systematic review and meta-analysis', *Journal of the American Medical Association*, 2013

Friedman, Jeffrey, 'A war on obesity, not the obese', *Science,* February 2003

Griffiths, C, Gately, P, Marchant, PR and Cooke, CB, 'Area-level deprivation and adiposity in children: is the relationship linear?', *International Journal of Obesity*, April 2013

Howard, BV, Manson, JE, Stefanick, ML, Beresford, SA, Frank, G, Jones, B, Rodabough, RJ, Snetselaar, L, Thomson, C, Tinker, L, Vitolins, M, Prentice, R, 'Low-fat dietary pattern and weight change over seven years: the Women's Health Initiative Dietary Modification Trial', *Journal of the American Medical Association*, January 2006

Jebb, Susan et al, 'Primary care referral to a commercial provider for weight loss treatment versus standard care: a randomised controlled trial', *Lancet*, October 2011

Jeffery, Alison et al., 'Parents' awareness of overweight in themselves and their children: cross-sectional study within a cohort' (EarlyBird 21), *British Medical Journal*, December 2004

Johnson, F, Cooke, L, Croker, H, Wardle, J, 'Changing perceptions of weight in Great Britain: comparison of two population surveys', *British Medical Journal*, July 2008

Jones Nielsen, Jessica, 'Rising obesity-related hospital admissions among children and young people in England: national time trends study', *PLOS One*, June 2013

Katan, Martijn B, 'Weight-loss diets for the prevention and treatment of obesity', *New England Journal of Medicine*, February 2009

Leibel RL, Rosenbaum M, and Hirsch J, 'Changes in energy expenditure resulting from altered body weight', *New England Journal of Medicine*, August 1995

Lissner, Lauren, Odell, Patricia M, D'Agostino, Ralph B, Stokes, Joseph III, Kreger, Bernard, Belanger, Albert J, Brownell, Kelly D, 'Variability of body weight and health outcomes in the Framingham population', *New England Journal of Medicine*, June 1991

Lustig, Robert H, Schmidt, Laura A, Brindis, Claire D, 'Public health: the toxic truth about sugar', *Nature*, February 2012

Mann, Traci, Tomiyama, A Janet, Westling, Erika, Lew, Ann-Marie, Samuels, Barbra, Chatman, Jason, 'Medicare's search for effective obesity treatments: diets are not the answer', *American Psychologist,* April 2007

Mattison, J et al, 'Impact of calorie restriction on health and survival in rhesus monkeys from the NIA study', *Nature,* September 2012

Muennig, P et al, 'I think therefore I am: perceived ideal weight as a determinant of health', *American Journal of Public Health,* March 2008

Padwal, Raj S, Pajewski, Nicholas M, Allison, David B, Sharma, Arya M, 'Using the Edmonton obesity staging system to predict mortality in a population-representative cohort of people with overweight and obesity', *Canadian Medical Association Journal,* August 2011

Perez-Pastor, E et al, 'Assortative weight gain in mother-daughter and father-son pairs: an emerging source of childhood obesity', *International Journal of Obesity,* July 2009

Piernas, Carmen and Popkin, Barry, 'Trends in snacking among US children', *Health Affairs,* 2010

Pomeranz, J and Rutkow, L., 'Efforts to immunize food manufacturers from obesity-related lawsuits: a challenge for public health', *Corporations and Health Watch,* August 2011

Rayner, Geof and Lang, Tim, 'Is nudge an effective public health strategy to tackle obesity? No', *British Medical Journal,* April 2011

Rolls, Barbara, 'Sensory-specific Satiety', *Nutrition Reviews,* April 2009

Singhal, Atul and Lucas, Alan, 'Early origins of cardiovascular disease: is there a unifying hypothesis?', *Lancet,* May 2004

Stuckler, David and Nestle, Marion, 'Big food, food systems, and global health', *PLOS Medicine,* June 2012

Sumithran, P et al, 'Long-term persistence of hormonal adaptations to weight loss', *New England Journal of Medicine,* October 2011

Swinburn, Boyd, 'The global obesity pandemic: shaped by global drivers and local environments', *Lancet,* August 2011

Te Morenga, L, Mallard, S, Mann, J, 'Dietary sugars and body weight: systemic review and meta-analyses of randomised controlled trials and cohort studies', *British Medical Journal,* January 2013

Uauy, Ricardo, 'Do we believe Derek's motives for taking his new job at PepsiCo?', *Public Health Nutrition,* February 2008

Viner, Russell, Roche, Edna, Maguire, Sabine, Nicholls, Dasha, 'Childhood protection and obesity: framework for practice', *British Medical Journal,* July 2010

Wagner, B et al, 'Extreme obesity is associated with suicidal behaviour and suicide attempts in adults: results of a population-based representative sample', *Depression and Anxiety,* October 2013

INDEX